"Heather has laid out the road map over fifty-two weeks to help you create your own healthy lifestyle that works for you and one to get excited about because it's not daunting. You'll feel in control yet relaxed, inspired, and ready to take actionable steps to find the happiest healthiest you that has always been there. You've got this, and Heather will steer you in the right direction!"

—Joy McCarthy, certified nutritionist
and three-time best-selling cookbook author

"As a clinical nutritionist for forty years I have been a longtime fan of Heather's knowledge, enthusiasm, and caring for the quality health of people. Read her words and listen carefully; she has a wealth of information that is needed by all of us. If you eat and breathe, Heather can help!"

—Freddy S. Kaye, PhD, LD, clinical nutritionist

"None of us can go it alone, and Heather Fuselier is a cheerful, gifted, compassionate, and entertaining companion on your road to wellness. Wherever you are on your journey—even if you haven't found the starting line yet—*Happy, Healthy You* will give you practical tools and useful insights into your lifelong patterns and how to create new, better ones. Fuselier has a refreshingly frank take on self-awareness that has persuaded even this cynical journalist to give happiness a try."

—Randi Atwood, *USA Today* Network—Florida

HEATHER FUSELIER

happy, healthy
you

BREAKING THE RULES
FOR A WELL-BALANCED LIFE

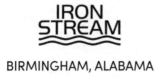

IRON
STREAM

BIRMINGHAM, ALABAMA

Happy, Healthy You

Iron Stream
An imprint of Iron Stream Media
100 Missionary Ridge
Birmingham, AL 35242
IronStreamMedia.com

Library of Congress Control Number: 2022930780

Cover design by Hannah Linder Designs

ISBN: 978-1-64526-356-2 (paperback)
ISBN: 978-1-64526-357-9 (e-book)

1 2 3 4 5—26 25 24 23 22

For my dad, my original inspiration

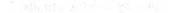

Contents

Contents

Introduction

I'm so glad you're here.

This book is for you—all of you. The part of you that is motivated to do big, bold things, the part of you that isn't, the part of you that wonders what it will take to finally make life changes stick, and the part of you that just wants to take a nap and wake up with all your problems solved.

As a national board-certified health and wellness coach, I've helped hundreds of people break out of that frustrating stop-start cycle and commit to accomplishing their goals. In this book, I'll guide you through the steps to become your own partner and create a lifestyle that supports your best life. After all, before you can be yourself, you need to know yourself.

In this fifty-two-week guide, you'll discover a healthy lifestyle that fits your needs. Each entry includes a story, followed by a practical "While We're on the Subject," a "Make Your Own Rules" weekly assignment or recommended focus, and questions for reflection or journaling.

We're surrounded by messages telling us to live confidently, think positively, follow our bliss, end toxic relationships, practice self-care, and let it all go. This book gives you a road map to reach those aspirations.

The healthy living to-do list is short and simple. Eat healthy, exercise, get to bed on time, and don't stress. But knowing and doing are different. Relax. Help is here. Explore how to understand your values and priorities, set boundaries, create a vision for your life, and enjoy it now.

Lessons from a Race Car Driver

My friend hired someone to work in his mechanic shop.

The new hire had spent the bulk of his career as a race car driver, a profession that seems to add electricity to a conversation. A race car driver? Not someone you meet every day. I visualized a huddle of middle-aged men recalling their glory days. Their eyes twinkled as they angled for stories from the pit, transported to their boyhood fascination with the roar of an engine. (Girls love cars, too, but in this case, it was boys.)

Eventually my friend explained to me how he came to hire the race car driver in the first place. Turns out that drag racing was too rough on the man's body. "Even with all the modern technology in cars these days?" the other men asked. "Even with all the padding and reinforced clothing drivers wear?"

"Yes," my friend continued. "Driving the car was no problem at all. Stopping, however, was a different story."

"Stopping," the race car driver said, "put me in retirement."

When my friend reached this part of the story, I pulled out my notebook because he had given me something to think about.

Stopping had been hard on the driver's body because of the tremendous jolt his body received when the parachute suddenly popped out behind him—even though he was expecting it. The latest, greatest technology can only do so much in a war with physics. Over time, the residual effects of that impact on the man's body became more trouble than thrill, and he retired. In a sense, stopping over and over again forced him into retirement.

How often do we speed through life until something stops us—a family crisis, an illness, a job loss, or some other game-changer. Those events don't usually allow for gradual decelerations that gently and safely roll us into a new destination. No, game-changing events come with skid marks, screeching tires, and all manner of chaos. In my line of work, that kind of sudden impact translates to more fast-food meals, more missed workouts, and more sleepless nights. When your healthy habits come to a screeching halt, your body feels the impact. Keep up that cycle long enough and your health will deteriorate.

But what if the driver had kept speeding around the track and never stopped? He wouldn't have felt the impact of continual stops and wouldn't have needed to retire. Tempting, yes, but we know that's not a plausible answer. Eventually, he would run out of gas, the tires would shred, and the engine would dry up. Never stopping isn't the solution either.

You know the answer, don't you? Of course you do. Maintain a consistent, slower speed so when the need arises, changing course doesn't mean slamming on the brakes and jolting everything. Yeah, that's the same slow-and-steady healthy-living advice dressed up in a new way.

Here are some ways you can implement the advice this week:

- In your "diet starts tomorrow" zeal, you may be tempted to commit to rising early each morning to go to the gym, exercise, and maybe even enroll in a ninety-day fitness challenge to motivate yourself to get in shape. Whoa! Too fast. Three to four challenging workouts per week are more manageable and less likely to result in burnout or injury.
- You may be ready to purge the pantry and fridge of all temptation, buy the latest diet book, adopt your ancestors' culinary habits, and never eat carbohydrates again. Watch out! You're going to crash. Lightening up your favorite

recipes and eating out less often is a clear path to progress and easier to maintain, especially if you still want a social life.

Here's the truth: life is going to happen, and you'll need to course-correct. If you're careening around the curve at top speed trying to do the extreme version of your healthy goals, you'll crash and be unable to drive again for a while. That would be a shame, considering how much work you did to establish a healthier routine.

So, take a lesson from the driver. Constantly stopping and starting took such a toll on him that he couldn't race anymore. When you slide into the driver's seat of your healthy goals, drive slowly. Sure, maintaining a steady pace isn't as thrilling or exciting as taking the curves at top speed, but you can drive the car a lot longer.

While We're on the Subject . . .

I used to think I didn't have time to nap, but that's because I didn't know how to do it. Yes, as elementary as it sounds, napping as adults is a skill we may need to relearn.

All naps are not created equal. Duration affects the benefits. When I gained a better understanding of naps, I gained a new appreciation for them. I now take power naps when my schedule permits, and I've been surprised how energetic and creative I feel after the right nap.

If you're ready to learn how to take a good nap, follow these general guidelines:

- Twenty-five minutes boosts alertness and motor learning skills.
- Forty-five minutes boosts memory and enhances creativity.
- Seventy-five minutes enhances problem-solving skills.

Make Your Own Rules

Choose three to four challenging workouts to make a part of your weekly routine. If you already have a workout plan, you may need to cut it down to whatever feels manageable. Also, plan your meals for this week, allowing space for new, healthy recipes as well as some of your favorite not-so-healthy recipes.

Reflect

1. Recall a time when your healthy intentions were interrupted by external factors. What factors tend to get in the way of creating a healthy routine?
2. Based on your current abilities and experience with exercise, what two simple changes can you make to the workout schedule (or lack thereof) you currently follow?
3. Based on your dietary habits and needs, what two simple changes can you make to your diet this week?

WEEK 2

Adjust Expectations for a Healthy Weekend

One Friday evening, my friend blew into the restaurant like a hurricane. She collapsed into a chair, dropped her phone into the overflowing bag on the seat next to her, and grabbed a menu. "Finally, Friday! It's my cheat meal, so I can eat whatever I want!" She then ordered something she considered indulgent and satisfying.

As she ate her reward for being good all week, I thought about the pendulum she clung to, swinging from closely monitoring her nutrition and meals during the week to eating whatever she desired in whatever amount she desired on the weekend. Was she enjoying the ride or hanging on for dear life?

I've done both. I suspect you have as well.

My clients often tell stories of being good during the week and bad on the weekends. Not too long ago, my weekends felt like that too. I was continually ticked off that I always seemed to take three steps forward, then two steps back.

Weekends are a notoriously difficult time to stick to a healthy routine. The weekend begs for a break from the norm. But if you're working hard to decrease your health risks, consistency over the weekend can move you forward to the next level. Over time, I've created several strategies to hurdle the weekend and land on Monday feeling much, much better.

Decide What You Want. Yes, you choose! When you look forward to your weekend, how do you want to feel at the end—energized, relaxed, rejuvenated, prepared? Put some adjectives on your mood for Sunday night, then consider what needs to happen on Friday and Saturday to feel that way on Sunday. Also consider what should not happen. You know what I'm talking about.

Adjust the Dial. Once you've chosen a desired outcome, look at the big picture and determine how realistic that outcome is, based on what you're willing to do or not do. Some clients set a goal of drinking less beer on the weekend. Drinking no beer isn't usually realistic, but a goal of drinking less beer is. Be honest with yourself about what a realistic outcome means for you, then adjust the dial to a goal that represents progress without swinging the pendulum too far.

Do a Gut Check. Any good wellness coach will challenge you to go deep. Why is this outcome important to you? Why do you want to change your weekends? What will you miss out on if you don't change? What will you gain if you work hard for change this time? Outcomes are important because when the going gets tough, you'll need a reason that pulls at you.

Clear the Obstacles. Make it easier to achieve your goal by removing the obstacles. If your goal is to maintain good nutrition, keep as many of your weekend meals the same as your weekday meals as possible, and log them in advance in a calorie tracker such as MyFitnessPal. This gives you an opportunity to see potential slip points and plan for them ahead of time. Other tips:

- If you're going to a restaurant, read the menu online and decide what to order before you arrive. At the restaurant, order first before you lose your resolve and get sucked in by other people's selections.

- Work out on the weekend. Starting the day with exercise helps curb your appetite for splurges and revs up your metabolism.
- Chop fruits and veggies for snacks all at once or buy them pre-chopped. Grabbing prepared snacks out of the fridge is easier than taking out a piece of fruit, a knife, and a cutting board.
- Put a white board on your fridge and write out your menu for the weekend. Seeing it in black and white will not only keep you organized but also serve as extra accountability when you open that door and grab a snack.
- Don't buy junk. If it's not there, you won't eat it. And don't say you're buying it for the kids or your spouse or whatever. They don't need junk food either.

Be Loud and Proud. Sharing your intention to be healthy over the weekend with a buddy, family member, or random people at the coffee café gives you extra accountability and makes you feel more in charge of your weekend. Plus, you may inspire a friend to join you, and then you can keep each other honest. Here are some ways to voice this goal:

- Keep it positive. Focus on what you're doing for yourself (having a healthy weekend), not what you're missing (I'm skipping dessert).
- Keep it present tense. Talking about being healthy in the future is fine, but the difference between "I'm having a healthy weekend" and "I'm going to have a healthy weekend" can be huge. The word *tomorrow* can be added to the second statement way too easily.

Keep in mind that a cheat day only cheats you. You deserve better. You work hard all week to establish healthy behaviors and fuel your body, and you can take it to the next level when you maintain consistency over the weekend. Decide what you want, remove the barriers, and jump off the weekend pendulum.

While We're on the Subject . . .

Write down your current habits in terms of exercise, eating, stress, and rest. Then set one or two manageable goals for each of these categories. At the end of the week, reassess and determine whether you should adjust your goals to fit a more realistic lifestyle.

Make Your Own Rules

Pay attention to where your mind wanders this week. When it wanders, take note of the scenario in your head. Assess whether that distraction is something you truly desire or only a fleeting thought. Are you willing to do what's necessary to attain that dream, or is it just something fun to think about? Do this every time you notice your mind wandering.

Reflect

1. Do you notice any patterns in your mind-wandering? What themes or scenarios do you often find yourself imagining?
2. What would your life look like if you pursued your most significant and provoking thought about improving your life?
3. Have you ever taken action on a daydream? What made that possible?

WEEK 3

You Are Here

A recent conversation with a client went downhill quickly.

First, we talked about her weight loss goal and what she had been doing to achieve it. Our focus then shifted to her busy work schedule, then her son's upcoming wedding in another state. Soon we were anticipating what her future might look like, the medical woes of various family members, her own aching foot, and whether she should purchase a treadmill or a gym membership.

After a bit, I raised my hand and asked, "Where are we right now?" I'd been so caught up in the stories that I wasn't sure if we were still talking about what we had met to discuss—her weight loss goal.

Imagine you're in a crowded shopping mall where every corridor looks the same. A stranger stops you and asks, "Is there a place nearby to eat?" Bewildered, you look around and think, *I don't even know where I am.* So, the two of you look for one of those maps—the kind with an arrow that points to your location and says, "You are here." Then things start to make sense again. You figure out where the other person needs to go and the best way to get there. Everything feels better.

My client's path to a healthier self needed that kind of map. She and I needed to stop, back up, and look for the arrow that says, "You are here," so we could get our bearings.

And that's what we did. We pulled out a blank piece of paper and drew a map of where she was and where she wanted to go. In between the start and finish points, we noted all the other stuff that had distracted us and caused us to get lost in the first place so she could navigate around them. With the map in hand, the way forward became much clearer.

Have you ever been lost? Have you ever felt like you've fallen so far down the rabbit hole of healthy gimmicks that you can't find your way back to where you started? I've been there, and being lost wasn't fun. My choices didn't seem to matter because I was going in circles anyway. When you realize you're lost, the best option is to stop and figure out where you are. If that sounds easier said than done, here's a hint: you are where you are. That's the only place you can be, so that part is easy.

The next part takes a little imagination. Mentally zoom out from where you are and imagine your life as a big map. Look off to the right, and you may imagine something that represents your destination. In my mind, I see a red blinking button flashing, "Look! Over here!"

Next, forget the reasons you got lost and look for the most direct path to your destination, your goal. You are here, you want to go there, and here's the straight line to get there.

Now, take note of your predictable roadblocks. The life stuff that gets in the way. I know, you think those issues won't come up this time, but they have a sneaky way of showing up right when you don't expect them. Be prepared.

You're now ready to travel again. You have your map, you know where you're going, and you're aware of what could block your path. Down the road, if you feel lost again, pull out the map and ask yourself, "Where am I?"

Life is a series of course corrections; we're all traveling that road together. Zoom out, get your bearings, and make sure you're still headed in the right direction.

While We're on the Subject . . .

One day when I was at the playground with one of my kids, an ant crawled over my leg. I watched it walk around, eventually move to a leaf, and then crawl on some mulch. I studied its legs, its segmented body, and all its bits and parts. I didn't know that was a form of meditation. I definitely felt more relaxed and less distracted when I snapped out of my Zen-ant moment, but I didn't make the connection until I read about flower meditation.

In flower meditation, you examine all the parts of a flower: the curves, textures, colors, and anything else you observe. Meditation and mindfulness go hand in hand. When sitting in silence and focusing on your breath isn't your jam, focusing on the minute details of a flower might be. I have one suggestion— start small. Even a few minutes of meditation can make a big difference.

Make Your Own Rules

Draw a map to guide you toward your desired destination. Write down where you are and where you want to be, then fill in the possible roadblocks. Finish by mapping the most direct route from your current location to your destination.

Reflect

1. Where are you right now? Where do you want to be?
2. What obstacles may prevent you from reaching your desired destination?
3. What distractions draw your attention away from the pursuit of your goal?

WEEK 4

Control-Alt-Delete

As I wrote an email, my computer screen froze—something for which I had no patience. I was already annoyed with the computer's pop-up window about installing updates when I was clearly working on something important. After my usual technical troubleshooting strategies failed—clicking the mouse a bunch of times in a row, then moving it all around my mouse pad—I moved to my ultimate defense tactic: simultaneously pressing Control-Alt-Delete.

Most people who use Microsoft Windows know that when you deploy the Control-Alt-Delete maneuver, a pop-up window appears that gives you the power to make your computer stop doing something you don't like. But on this day, my computer ignored me. So, I tried again: Control-Alt-Delete. Still, I was denied.

As I placed my fingers on the keys and said aloud, as if that made a difference, "Control, Alt, Delete," the irony was obvious. Not only had my computer chosen to install updates at an inconvenient time, but it was also freezing up and forcing me to take control, make alterations, and if necessary, delete.

A lot like life, right? We're three weeks into our healthy habits commitment, so the grand promises we made about lifestyle changes have reached a point of reckoning. We're happy about some new routines we've adopted. Other habits are a little harder to maintain, but they're coming along. And some of us feel like our new routine is trying to install updates in our life when we're still trying to hit Send on our previous lifestyle. Is that happening to you? Take control, alter things, and if necessary, delete.

Here are some ideas to help you make that happen.

Assess What You Can Control. The best goals are grounded in what we can do on our own. Do you have a goal that depends on someone else? Is a lack of progress frustrating because you're waiting for a phone call or decision before you take the next step? Fretting over what disrupts our environment and leaves us without recourse is human, but rushing around to confirm that those aggravations are still there is a waste of energy. Focus instead on what you can control—how you react, how you manage the stress of waiting, and the positive steps you can take on your own. Let go of the rest.

Alter What You Can. Releasing control doesn't mean washing your hands of anything that doesn't fit your worldview. Sometimes what seems out of your control is more manageable than you think. What can be altered? If the new workout routine isn't doable, consider another time of day or location. If the weekly healthy grocery shopping becomes burdensome, why not make several small trips instead of one big one? Step back from what you think is unchangeable and see whether the pieces can fit together in a different way.

Delete What Isn't Working. Imagine a crowd of people behind you holding the other end of rubber bands attached to your arms, legs, waist, and feet. Now imagine trying to take a step forward and another and another. As more people or obligations grab the rubber bands, the weight of them stops your progress. But if you reach back and cut some of those rubber bands, you can move forward more easily.

As a working mom trying to strike a balance between taking care of everyone and having a life of my own, I seem to add a new rubber band every week. But I also delete some: the to-do items I carry over from week to week without much consequence are the first to go. The events I keep missing clearly are not priorities; they are deleted for now. Assess what you can realistically delete so you can move forward on what matters. Even one or two deletions may make a difference.

On the day my computer was so uncooperative, I eventually fixed the problem. I turned the computer off and back on again, which is the computer equivalent to deep breathing and a stretch. When my internet browser reopened and asked if I wanted to restore all the windows that were open before the computer shut down, I chose to start over fresh.

Sometimes what's going on isn't working, so take control of the situation, alter and delete what you can, then focus on what's most important.

While We're on the Subject . . .

Regularly remind yourself of the difference between what you can and can't control. When I was young, my mom often advised me not to worry about situations I couldn't control. In my cocky youth, I thought I could control anything if I worked hard enough. Right? Wrong. Accepting that I couldn't control situations even if I worked hard was discouraging. Isn't everything possible with hard work and perseverance?

There is good news, of course. A third category exists: situations that can happen and I'll still be OK. That list developed over time, but I'm learning that in plenty of circumstances, I don't need to react at all.

Accept that some parts of life are allowed to exist without you forming an opinion about them. How much energy would you save if you let them go? How much energy would be freed up for fun activities, for creative thinking, and for peace of mind?

I know what you're thinking. Not everything is OK, Heather. I know, but that's OK too. With patience and practice, when those events come up, you'll be able to tell the difference between what needs your attention and what doesn't.

Make Your Own Rules

Instead of categorizing events by whether or not you're in control, let them be in the third column. Then, when they happen, just say, "OK" or "great." Or nothing.

Reflect

1. What do you really need to be in control of?
2. What can be changed, moved, or modified so it's a better fit for your life?
3. What could be deleted and no one would notice?

WEEK 5

Take Your Next Best Opportunity

Are you an optimist or a pessimist? Optimistic thinking leads to resilience, positive outcomes, and even a healthier brain and body. But this week, I'm encouraging you to go a different way. I want you to think about the worst-case scenario.

Don't worry. We won't stay here long. But for a minute or two, think of the ways your healthy plans could be derailed this week. Indulge your inner curmudgeon and let him point out all the flaws in your plan. Rain on your parade. Ready? Go.

OK, now put on your optimist hat. Acknowledge the potential ways your plans could go awry, then go forth. *Carpe diem!* Seize the day. March into the day knowing your plans may go wrong, but you're committed to move forward anyway.

In the past, I used the list of what could go wrong as a starting point for negotiations between my present and future self. For example, I may allow my present self to have an extra slice of pizza in exchange for my future self getting up and running the next morning to burn it off. Sound familiar? How about eating all the cookies today because tomorrow you're giving them up and will never eat them again? Or going out for a last meal before your diet begins? Yep, we've all been trapped by the diet mentality, convinced that if we can have what we want right now (give in to the pessimist), surely we'll happily comply with the consequences later (believe the optimist).

Except that I might hit snooze on the alarm too many times the next morning and never make time for that run. Or other circumstances might arise that make it impossible to select the healthy choice—or if not impossible, then definitely less fun and better off postponed to a day better suited for the straight and narrow. Like Monday. Nothing wipes the slate clean like the promise of doing better tomorrow.

The truth is that healthy habits are a zero-sum game that starts with a fresh scoreboard every day. We can't go back and fix what happened yesterday. Sorry to say this, friends, but a healthy lifestyle is a daily gig. There are no breaks.

But that's OK. Set aside whatever reasons the pessimist created and focus on making today the best day possible given the circumstances. Seizing the day for better health doesn't necessarily mean making the most of every opportunity. The secret is staying upright no matter what tries to knock you down. Truly seizing the day means walking into the wind, knowing you can make the day great even if it wasn't what you hoped for.

Stop bargaining with yourself with the expectation that you can fix the situation tomorrow. Don't save up calories, don't burn them in advance, don't do something today anticipating something else later. Make today healthy because you deserve to feel great today. Tomorrow, make the same commitment to yourself. And again. And again. Sure, some days are better than others. Don't worry about that. Seize today, give it your best effort, and the big goal will take care of itself.

To fully embrace the practice of *carpe diem*, celebrate each effort and every victory along the way. A morning habit of writing down your intentions sets a positive tone, and a nightly gratitude journal offers a chance to reflect on your progress. Acknowledge what you could have done better, then frame that goal as an opportunity instead of a punishment.

I imagine that when the Roman poet Horace suggested *carpe diem*, he had a sense of urgency about the human spirit and didn't want us to miss opportunities because we were worrying about the future. This week, face into the wind and go forward with enthusiasm and curiosity about how you're going to stay upright.

While We're on the Subject . . .

During a bout of organizing, I found a vision board that I'd made a couple of years earlier. I enjoy creating vision boards because the process allows me to think through my aspirations, evaluate what they require of me, and be inspired by the pictures and words I choose to represent them.

In this case, finding the vision board was extra fun because I realized that I've achieved a good bit of what's on it, even if not in the way I expected. Pretty cool!

One of the defining elements of my vision board was this quotation by Oprah Winfrey: "The real point of being alive is to evolve into the whole person you were intended to be."[1] I liked her perspective, so I tacked it up. A few days later, I walked past my vision board, propped up on the mirror above my dresser, and the word *evolve* jumped out at me. Hmph, I thought. Who has time to evolve? I want life to be the way I want it now. But I knew that word was important, so I picked up a pen and circled it.

At my computer, I looked up the definition of *evolve* and smirked when I saw that the Latin root is *evolvere*, which means "to unroll." Of course.

When something evolves, it changes. It grows—morphs, adapts, streamlines, becomes something new—through its experiences. We can't rush evolution. Creating change in our lives, especially how we manage our health and well-being, is also a process. Although thinking about changing the course of our lives and everything that entails can be overwhelming, change can also be calm and steady if we allow ourselves to unroll slowly.

In a world that promises results in ninety days and praises overnight success stories, waiting to evolve into the person you were intended to be seems like sitting on the sidelines. We're supposed to make it happen. Just do it! Be the change you want to see in the world. *Carpe diem.* And hurry!

We want to force change, so we keep shoving it into place, as if we're trimming the ends of life's puzzle pieces so they fit together into something that might stay that way, as long as no one touches it. But then life buckles and warps, and the pieces come apart, and we know we should have slowed down and let life unroll at its own pace.

Make Your Own Rules

Be Proactive about Change. Evolution favors the proactive: those who are willing participants in the process of being changed and open to the possibility that rolling with change may send them in a better direction than they planned. Create a vision for how you want to live your life and manage your health, set your course for that destination, and launch that ship, friend. Go for it.

Respond. This is the key element of evolving into the person you were intended to be: notice when you have to keep shoving those pieces back in place and respond to that. If sticking to your charted course requires a rigid lifestyle that can't be maintained without constant attention, you're probably headed in the wrong direction. Healthy changes may be difficult, but they are attainable when they're also sustainable. Pay attention and respond.

Take the Steps. The balance between proactive and responsive is partnership. Changing all your habits at once in pursuit of a healthier life isn't realistic or practical but taking the first step is doable. Relax. Don't rush the process. Allow yourself to unroll and evolve into the person you are intended to be by taking the next positive step toward your goal.

Reflect

1. Taking the first step requires bravery. What words do you associate with being brave?
2. Whose bravery and willingness to seize the day do you admire?
3. What would you do today if you knew you could handle the outcome regardless of what it is? (Do it!)

WEEK 6

Create Your Favorite Life

Imagine you hold a ball of yarn that represents time. On one side of your body sits a pile of unraveled yarn that signifies the amount of time that passed before you were born, the millions of years that occurred before you got here—the people and the dinosaurs and the plate tectonics and everything that happened before us. On the other side of your body is the rest of the ball of yarn, representing the time yet to come. In front of your body is a span of yarn about two feet long, which signifies the average human lifespan of seventy-nine years. One side is millions of years, one side is infinity, and in the middle is your lifespan.

Seventy-nine years is not very long when compared to time past and time future. Some of us have longer lifespans, some shorter. When we break life down into childhood, adolescence, and adulthood, the span seems even shorter. At the beginning, all we can do is kid stuff, and we have to obey grown-ups. Then come the teen years when a lot of us act like idiots, and then comes a decent span when we mostly have life together. But even then, what we're really living for is retirement, when we can jump off the job treadmill and do whatever we want. After a few years of retirement, our health may fail, then we die.

To maximize this short life, a health movement began with the goal of living your best life. Books, blogs, podcasts, magazines, and television shows were launched to help us learn how to become our absolute best and suck the marrow out of every day.

Carpe diem! Bucket lists. Make the most of every moment. We chase this ideal, thinking that being the best version of ourselves will mean we lived life more fully, that we didn't waste any time. But pursuing the ideal is a good way to miss our life because we spend most of our time striving to be our best self. Instead, we should be our favorite self.

Your favorite self might not be your best self. Your potential is unlimited, so who determines when you have become your best? We can always improve on what we've done, so striving to be our best seems kind of exhausting.

Busy people often say that good is the enemy of great, but good is not the enemy of great. Good is fantastic, and good is satisfying. Instead of living your best life, I invite you to live your favorite one. Why? When you're connected to something that brings you joy—the job you wish you had, the work you would do for free—that joy cannot be hidden. It radiates from you to others in a significant way.

When you're connected to a purpose, you infect others with that same passion. Just the fact that you're living your favorite life energizes others to do the same. People who shape their lives around their purpose are more productive, less stressed out, less likely to engage in addictive behaviors, and more likely to increase their lifespan.

What was that? You heard me.

How do you tell the difference between your best life and your favorite life? Here's a clue: your best life has a much longer to-do list, and your favorite life can be satisfied with much less. These ideas may help you discover your favorite life:

- When you notice that you're smiling in a genuine, natural way, take some notes. What makes you smile? Look beyond what's visible to what that smile represents.
- Ask others what you are good at. When others ask you to do or teach something, why do they choose you?

- Listen to your rants. What gets you fired up? When you rant and rave, listen to yourself. What are you advocating for? Why is that important enough for you to shout?

Then let the rest go. Cull the to-do list that's taking up your precious life and delete the optional items that aren't connected to your purpose. You'll learn to discern what to let go and what to keep by how you feel when it happens.

Life is short. Life is good. This week when you catch yourself smiling, I hope you feel good enough to let the rest go.

While We're on the Subject . . .

No. Nope. No way. Not gonna happen. Negative. Forgot. Veto. Denied. Uh-uh.

The English language provides dozens of ways to say no, but for such a small word—just two letters—with so many variations, we have a hard time coming up with a way to say it without feeling uncomfortable.

After all, saying yes is often the fastest route to feeling less stress, because we know that's what others want. Saying no can increase stress and anxiety, induce feelings of guilt or shame, and lead to arguments and tension in relationships. But it doesn't have to. You can learn how to say no gracefully and positively, protecting your boundaries and health.

Know Your Boundaries. Helping people feels good, so set a certain amount of time you can give to others each week or month. Then honor that amount and only commit to what can be done in that amount of time—whether it's an hour a day or a weekend each month. Set boundaries for helping others as you would allot a specific amount of time for an appointment at work. After you reach the allotted limit, look forward to helping again next time.

Stop Apologizing. No is a complete sentence. You don't need to justify or explain why you can't commit. Practice a few positively phrased responses such as "That sounds like fun. I'm at my limit for now" or "Thank you for thinking of me. I can't help now, but I hope it goes well." Over time, others will respect and admire the honesty of your positive, balanced responses.

Focus on What You Can Do. Attending another office birthday party and want to avoid the cake? Bring a healthy snack for other like-minded teammates, keep a bottle of water in your hand, and keep smiling and talking. Reframing what may feel like a barrier ("I can't have cake") into an opportunity ("another chance to practice my mantra") can put the power and confidence back in your hands.

Make Your Own Rules

When you're surrounded by temptation and determined to maintain balance, a few trick phrases can be your secret weapon. A couple of my favorites are "I'm saying yes to me" and "This is temporary." Keep your mantra positive and focus on succeeding, not resisting. You'll leave that environment feeling successful rather than deprived and depleted.

Saying no can be liberating, powerful, and even help others by opening their eyes to new, creative alternatives. Learning to say no takes practice, so start with the small stuff as you build your confidence and comfort level. Before long, saying no will begin to feel like saying yes to yourself, leading you to greater levels of calmness, confidence, and the capacity to do your best work.

Reflect

1. When have you had to disappoint someone to stay true to yourself?
2. When have you said no and felt no regrets?
3. How can you make it easier for someone you love to live his or her favorite life?

WEEK 7

Use the Right Tool for Stress Relief

Some people are stressed out by the unknown. Others obsess over the known—or what they think they know based on experience. Some feel the stress building up when they see a certain person or arrive at a particular location. Some of us pretend that nothing bothers us, even though everyone else can plainly see we're wound tighter than a spring.

Do you know what kind of stress you have? Does identifying the cause matter?

Knowing the source of your stress can help you choose the best tool to manage it and, over time, learn how to reduce it. In-the-moment techniques such as deep breathing, a brisk walk, or using a meditation app can be effective for managing stress throughout the day, but if you're interested in digging a little deeper and being proactive about stress, consider which of the following categories best describe your stress and the responses that may alleviate it.

Avoidable Stress

Has anyone ever told you to get out of your own way? Maybe that person sees you making life more complicated than necessary through procrastination, poor time management, or inefficient patterns.

One day, in the drive-thru lane of a fast-food restaurant, I frantically tried to choose something healthy from the menu, feeling stress mount as my family grew impatient and the line of cars behind us got longer. That stress could've been avoided if I'd made myself a sandwich instead of relying on fast food. Now I don't leave for road trips without bringing along healthy snacks.

Sometimes you need to think more creatively. Break down the situation and identify precisely what's causing the stress. At the drive-thru, I felt rushed, and my food options were limited. Naming those feelings helped me choose the right solution.

To address avoidable stress, pay attention to the patterns of your agitation—time of day, type of circumstance, or group of people. Instead of expressing your stress, determine whether you can do anything to change the scenario in the future. Focus on what you can do, not what needs to be done by someone else. We'll talk more about that later.

Secondhand Stress

Imagine sitting in your office or your home. Someone enters the room with a big bucket and says, "I have a bunch of stress in here. Do you want some?" Then they dump it all on the floor.

This is secondhand stress—the stress that has nothing to do with us but comes into our space. This may be the friend who wants to tell you all about her family drama or a coworker who bursts into your office to vent about a situation you cannot address or solve.

Resist the temptation to roll around in that stress. Give people room to be grumpy, dramatic, or angry without absorbing their emotions. Recognizing that you are in a secondhand-stress situation will help you step away from it.

Underlying Stress

At times you may not be able to pinpoint what's causing stress. When stress becomes the new normal, the underlying cause may be unrelated to your current situation. Financial stress, troubled relationships, feeling unheard or unappreciated, or feeling resentful can prevent you from enjoying life's blessings because these circumstances keep stress at a constant hum.

You may need the guidance of a professional to resolve underlying stress. None of us can navigate life alone, especially the tough spots.

Unavoidable Stress

Family strain, medical diagnoses, the death of a loved one— these situations aren't our fault, but we still have to deal with them. Everyone does. In these times, call in those tried-and-true resilience tools such as deep breathing, yoga, meditation, and exercise. Some stress is unavoidable, but, thankfully, we also have tools that help us cope.

When stress bubbles up, put it in its place, then choose the best response and enjoy a quicker path to calmer days.

While We're on the Subject . . .

Did you know some foods can help relieve stress? No, not ice cream and chocolate. These stress-reducing foods provide nutrients that calm us, boost mental alertness, and reduce our blood pressure.

Nuts. Stress depletes our levels of Vitamin B, and nuts can help replace them. Nuts also reduce blood pressure thanks to a hearty dose of potassium. But watch the serving size—the calories in a handful of nuts adds up fast.

Avocados. Both a fruit and also a plant-based fat, avocados can build a stress barrier with the help of glutathione, a substance that specifically blocks intestinal absorption of certain fats that cause oxidative damage. Avocados also contain lutein, beta-carotene, vitamin E, and folate. Half an avocado diced on a salad or sliced on a sandwich elevates your lunch.

Chamomile Tea. Do you know why packages of tea bags feature relaxing pictures of flowers, meadows, and calm people? A study from the University of Pennsylvania showed a direct link between drinking chamomile tea daily and a significant drop in anxiety symptoms.[2]

Red Peppers. Dip slices of red pepper into hummus for an afternoon snack at work, and those budget worksheets may be easier to tackle. The high levels of vitamin C in red peppers reduce blood pressure and help us deal with stressful situations.

Spinach. Have you ever checked your magnesium levels? Low amounts of magnesium can cause stress and depression, and the dark green leaves of spinach can be the perfect antidote. Magnesium regulates cortisol and blood pressure and helps flush out the body when you're stressed. Including spinach, brown rice, beans, and other sources of magnesium in your meals can help you better manage the stress that comes your way.

Make Your Own Rules

Recognize these signals that your body is stressed out and needs a break:

- Low energy
- Headaches
- Upset stomach, including diarrhea, constipation, and nausea
- Aches, pains, and tense muscles
- Chest pain and rapid heartbeat
- Insomnia

- Frequent colds and infections
- Loss of sexual desire and/or ability

This week, keep a journal about the types of stress you experience, and try some of the responses mentioned above. Make a note of what works best.

Reflect

1. How do you know that you've hit the wall and need a break?
2. What's your usual go-to for stress relief, and what new stress buster do you want to try this week?
3. What can you do today to change your response when you notice you're stressed?

WEEK 8

Trade In Old Habits for New Ones

A few years ago, I purchased a new car. I wasn't very happy about it. My 2004 Subaru Forester and I had been together for thirteen years. Dented and faded, it rattled and made weird noises. My "I Love State Parks" bumper sticker was almost entirely worn off, and the car was missing nonessential parts I had ripped off on the side of the interstate so I could keep driving. But the Forester was paid for, it was cute, and it had a roof rack—which I never used but valued greatly. And I knew that car. We were a team. I could drive it with my eyes closed. (I did not do that.)

But change was inevitable. My Forester needed repairs more frequently, it was becoming inefficient, and after over a decade of use, well, let's just say it was tired. So, I bit the bullet and bought a Prius, which I enjoy driving even though I miss my clunky old car and grow nostalgic when I think of it.

Changing habits is like that sometimes, right? We've all accumulated certain habits over the years, and although we know they need to change and that we'll be happy with the outcome, we're cozy in our routine. Even if some habits are destructive, expensive, unproductive, and sometimes dangerous, we stick with them because they're familiar. Change involves risk—even when we believe the outcome will be good, even when the only risk is the possibility of feeling weird and mildly inconvenienced.

Well, guess what? No one ever said you couldn't be wistful for the old days. Changing habits doesn't necessarily mean closing a life door and pretending those practices never existed. You can change your health habits without saying goodbye to the way life used to be. These approaches to change may ease your transition.

Press Pause. When ending one habit and beginning another feels overwhelming, don't pressure yourself to cut ties. Just press Pause on unproductive routines—being too sedentary, eating too much, wasting time—and reserve the option to return to previous habits if the new ones don't work out. I haven't met anyone yet who wanted to go back to being sedentary, overeating, and wasting time. Don't worry about ending something. Just begin something else.

Let Yourself Mourn. If you're ready to close the door on a habit and never speak of it again, allow yourself time to mourn that loss. Yes, it's a loss! There is a win to everything we choose to do, whether or not the choice is healthy. When we choose to cook more instead of eating out, we lose the convenience of having someone else cook. Getting out of bed earlier to exercise means losing the coziness of blankets and pillows. Even our destructive habits have a beneficial element, so acknowledge what you're giving up to gain something else. That's fair. So be sad, then get yourself together and keep on keeping on.

Connect with the Payoff. The grief won't last long, I promise. Soon you'll like how your new habits make you feel, and the appeal of returning to old ones will fade. Acknowledge that truth and connect with it. Write the reasons you are happier in a notebook and refer to them from time to time. Jot down a challenge you overcame when reverting to old ways would have been easier. Keep a record of the payoffs—a smaller size of clothes, walking a flight of stairs without becoming winded, getting off medication—and read them. The more you connect with the benefits of your new choices, the less you'll feel tempted to look back.

But if you do look back, that's OK. I like heated seats, better fuel economy, an ice-cold air conditioner, and a warranty. Stylish and clean, my new Prius was the right choice. But that doesn't mean I don't sometimes miss the Forester. I'm not going back to it, but I can remember it with fondness.

Are you clinging to an old habit that's comfortable, easy, and familiar even though you know an upgrade makes sense? Shop around this week. Take new habits on a test drive. And when you're ready, press Pause or trade in the old ones for something new. That new-life smell is pretty sweet.

While We're on the Subject . . .

Running with my friends one day, I noted that the trees in the neighborhoods would soon lose their dead leaves and we'd see more wildlife walking around in the green spaces. At least I hoped we would.

Have you ever seen one thing more clearly after something else has fallen away? Perhaps a few unproductive habits need to die in our lives so we can see better choices more clearly and focus on them.

Maybe the routines that keep us from connecting with ourselves on an authentic level are like leaves on the trees of our lives. Visualize the doubts, negative thoughts, excuses, uncertainties, and wounds from past failures—all the layers we wear for protection—as leaves that hide the trunk and the bare branches we'd be without them.

Imagine what would happen if those leaves fell to the ground.

Make Your Own Rules

Like leaves on a tree, the doubts, negative thoughts, excuses, uncertainties, and past wounds of our lives are temporary—here for a season and then ready to fall away so we can start anew.

Do you need to shed some leaves? Perhaps some of your old habits don't serve a purpose anymore. Maybe you cling to a familiar litany of reasons you can't take the next step. Let those leaves fall. If you don't want to discard them, remind yourself: the change is only for a season.

Leaves always return. In the spring, green shoots emerge and become new leaves that will also be shed when their productivity ends. And between seasons, you'll have time to savor the beauty of your bare branches and the strength of your trunk. The dead weight will be gone, and you can be . . . you.

Reflect

1. What could you see if you let the leaves of doubt fall?
2. What could you see if you let the leaves of negative self-talk fall?
3. What could you see if you let the leaves of excuses fall?

WEEK 9

Now You Know

As a child of the '80s, I sat on the living room floor on Saturday mornings watching television—the activity twenty-first-century moms feel guilty about allowing their children do. My friends and I rotted our brains as we ate sugary cereal, then ran out to the backyard and practiced unsupervised backflips off the monkey bars.

But we survived, thanks to the public service announcements that reminded us of the perils of making poor choices later in life, empowering us with a star shooting across the screen and its tagline, "The More You Know."

The message that awareness leads to change is still with me as an adult. As a certified wellness coach, I encourage people to do the best they can with what they know, then when they know better, do better. Healthy living is a journey. We take what we learn along the way and use the accumulated knowledge to make better decisions as we go. That's how life works. None of us get it right on the first day, and all of us look back at some point, marvel at the changes, and maybe even shake our heads, chuckle, and say, "If I knew then what I know now . . ."

We didn't know, but we did the best with what we did know, and we did better the next time. That's progress; that's growth.

Thinking about growth led to thinking about the honeymoon period of a new job. You know what I'm talking about: the first few months when you're new and don't know all the unspoken rules and routines, and you apologize with a shrug and a smile for a while. Over time, though, your coworkers and superiors expect you to learn how to do your job. During your first year, you will experience a variety of situations for the first time, but you gradually learn the ropes and become proficient. If not, you may find yourself smiling and shrugging in a new workplace.

The same learning curve happens when we adopt healthy living habits. Like a new job, we don't just show up to our healthy new lifestyle and get to work as if we had been there for months. But you're not a complete newbie at life. I'm willing to bet you already know some things that can make the transition easier.

You know what your schedule is. You know which mornings are hectic and which evenings allow time for exercise. An annoying realization may have tiptoed through your brain and said, "Dang it, if I'm going to exercise, I'll have to get up earlier." The thought may linger in the back of your mind, but it's there. You know.

You also know what usually happens when you go to a restaurant. The menus haven't changed. A voice in your head says what you should order, but you ignore it and order something else. You may not know the absolute best meal to order from a nutritional perspective, but you know enough to select a healthier choice. You know more than you think you do.

You know what time the gym opens and where to find healthy food at the grocery store. Unless you're brand-new in town, you can rattle off at least three suitable locations for exercise in a ten-mile radius of your home. You know.

You've learned a lot in life, but you don't yet know why you haven't taken action on what you know. Are there gaps you need to fill? Maybe the new routine feels overwhelming. Maybe you have a lot going on right now and can't focus on anything new until life calms down. Evaluating that knowledge is important too.

Consider what you know and compare it to what you want. Look for connections between what you know and what you want, then choose the easiest opportunity to make progress.

Remember, progress isn't about doing everything right; it's about using what you've learned to make better choices.

Some say knowledge is power, but I disagree. Knowledge is only the potential for power; when you take action on what you know, you gain power. And now you know.

While We're on the Subject . . .

Taking action on what you know can be difficult. When you're stuck between knowing you should do something but not knowing what it is, here are some ways to get yourself going again.

- **Consider how change benefits you.** This might seem like a no-brainer, but sometimes you must write down the benefits to think through how life could be better when you take action.
- **Consider how staying the same benefits you.** Yes, sameness has benefits. If you don't change, you don't have to think of new ideas. You can also stay where you know what to expect, where you know the rules, and where life is easy. Well, except for the changes you desire.
- **Add it up.** Yes, a good old-fashioned list of pros and cons can help you see the disparity between what is and what can be. Challenge yourself to explore your resistance to change and pay attention to what you discover.

Make Your Own Rules

Once you've been honest with yourself about the costs and benefits of change, imagine you're giving advice to a friend. What would you say? Would you be encouraging and supportive, or would you remind your friend of all her failures? Is there anything you feel excited to try? Give yourself grace to be messy, knowing you can always go back and try again.

Reflect

1. What would you do if success was guaranteed?
2. When have you taken a brave step and your courage paid off?
3. Which of your strengths can help you get up if you fall?

WEEK 10

The Why Is Bigger Than the How

If I conducted a poll and asked folks how to live healthy lives, most people would know the correct answers. Eating healthy food, watching portion size, exercising regularly, and managing stress top the to-do list. We know that. The mechanics of healthy living are simple. But we also know that simple isn't necessarily easy.

Let's imagine a follow-up question to my poll: Why? We know the how, even if we don't do it, so why don't we? I predict a much wider range of answers to that question, varying from practical to personal. Each response would vary because the why has to click within us.

The why, of course, is motivation. Many people have a goal to live healthier hidden somewhere within them, and those who pursue it have decided the benefit outweighs the hassle. When push comes to shove, an internal dialogue convinces them to lace up their sneakers and exercise. A mental switch flips and moves their hand away from the chips and toward the bottle of water. A voice in their head urges them to turn down the second helping. That motivation is the answer to their why.

Everyone's motivation is different, but some similarities emerge. A longer lifespan to enjoy grandchildren, improving mobility for an active retirement, getting off expensive medications, avoiding surgery, and increasing energy are some of the motivations I hear often. And if your motivation is to fit into your jeans and feel better when you look at vacation pictures, that's OK too. The more motivation you generate the better!

For me, the why comes in a combination of practicality and self-preservation. I have a busy schedule, and I know that if I don't exercise early in the morning, I'll run out of time and energy later in the day. When I plan and eat healthy meals, I feel my best. When I feel my best, stuff gets done. But when I skip my routine, I'm grumpy and disorganized. Adhering to my routine also helps me manage my weight. I remember how uncomfortable, tired, and frustrated I felt when I was overweight. I worked hard to lose weight, and I don't want to do that again. When that alarm goes off in the morning or I need to organize my meals for the next day, I don't debate how I will get out of bed or pack my lunch. I remind myself why. Sometimes I have to remind myself more than once, so my reasons to maintain my health goals need to be powerful enough to move me.

That's the key to healthy living. The reasons must be powerful enough to move you. Of all the perfectly logical reasons to eat healthy and exercise, only one or two may inspire you to get up and do something. Luckily, that's all you need. So how do you figure out what those motivations are?

The next time you're standing at a crossroads for your health, listen to the internal dialogue that takes place when you negotiate with yourself. Take a step back from yourself and be the judge and jury of your thoughts. Listen to your priorities debate and pay attention to which one wins. When you declare a winner, note the prevailing reason. There you have it: your true motivation.

If the healthy choice won, hooray! You're connected to a strong motivator (or have experienced the negative consequences enough times to know what's best for you). If other interests prevailed, be honest with yourself about why. Other priorities may take precedence over fitness. Maybe you don't take action because the goal has actually been set by someone else, and you resent it. Your awareness of the root motivator can relieve you from feeling like a failure for not reaching a goal you didn't set. Instead, negotiate new terms and establish a goal you care about.

Connect with your why this week. Put a picture of it on the fridge. Write it on your shoes. Tape it to your computer screen. Make it the ringtone on your phone. Do whatever's necessary to stay connected to your motivation. Because once you're connected with the why, the how becomes obvious.

While We're on the Subject . . .

Sometimes we aren't motivated to change until the situation has become so bad that the pain of change isn't as bad as the pain of staying the same. Other times we're more motivated by avoiding unsavory consequences than by the promise of a reward. That's OK. Your motivation isn't up for judgment or evaluation. No one else needs to know what it is.

Make Your Own Rules

Like trying to match wits with an insistent toddler, the word *why* can quickly become a maze of questions that leads you to places you never expected. Follow it. Keep asking yourself, "Why is this important? Why now? Why not wait?" The more connected you are to the benefits, the more easily you will create that reality.

Reflect

1. Why is now the right time to take that first brave step?
2. Have you ever used someone else's why as your motivation? How did that go?
3. How would you feel if you never achieved your dream?

WEEK 11

The War on Sugar Is All in Your Head

In the early years of my wellness coaching practice, before Americans became so aware of the sugar hidden in processed foods, many clients wanted help with beating what they considered an addiction to sugar.

I fielded many questions about sugar: how to break the habit, how to detect it in processed foods, and most frequently, which types are best or worst. "What about honey?" "Agave is better, right?" "Is Stevia better than Truvia?" "Does Splenda count as sugar?" The market was flooded with different versions and substitutes for the sweet stuff, each more exotic than the first, and I wondered if we were looking at the wrong part of the problem. After all, sugar has been around forever. It wasn't until we began using massive amounts of sugar to sweeten foods— virtually every processed food on the market—that sugar become a problem. The solution isn't connected to how gourmet or natural the sugar is because sugar isn't the problem. The problem is your response to any food that takes over your brain.

One of my clients had been sugar-free for a few months, and then she ate a holiday cookie and panicked. Fretting about her indiscretion, she confessed her sin to me and wrung her hands in despair. But as we talked about the incident, I learned that after eating the cookie she went about her life as normal. There was no landslide of overeating or binging on holiday sweets. She ate a cookie. "But I had sugar!" she cried. That's OK. The habit she'd broken three months previous was not about eating sugar; it was about changing her eating rituals. That's a bigger goal because those skills can be applied beyond sugar toward any out-of-control habit.

When we declare a personal war on sugar, we're battling our inability to live peacefully with it. Some say that sugar is an addiction, and at times it can certainly feel that way. But more addictive than the properties of any food are the rituals, behaviors, and traditions that accompany it. Any food eaten in secret, bought on the sly, used as a reward or stress buster, or eaten in shame is more toxic than any cookie. A plate of broccoli can be as dangerous as a bag of sugar if you can't stop eating it.

If your goal is to detox from sugar, congratulations. You're better off without it. But before you aim your arrow and declare war, make sure you're fighting the right battle.

While We're on the Subject . . .

Destructive patterns like emotional eating follow the same cycle as any other habit loop: the trigger, the response, and the reward. Sometimes avoiding the trigger is key to ending the cycle, but the next time you notice a craving for a habit you want to end, pay attention to how urgent the craving feels on a scale of one to five. Look around. What elements in your environment might be causing that effect? Do you see trends in the time of day, location, recent interactions, or work projects that could trigger the craving?

Make Your Own Rules

Do you want to decrease the amount of sugar in your diet? Pay extra attention for a couple of days to track how much sugar you eat on average and identify the easiest places to cut back, such as soda or juice drinks. Then select a few high-sugar foods to replace with lower-sugar alternatives. Finally, give your taste buds time to adjust. They need at least a couple of weeks to adapt to new flavors and appreciate the taste of food without added sugar. But they will adjust, and before long, you won't even notice the difference. I promise.

Reflect

1. What habits did you once wish to cultivate that are now part of your routine?
2. How did you develop these new habits?
3. What strengths help you sustain your new habits?

WEEK 12

The Social Side of Weight Loss

Growing up in the New Orleans area, I learned early that if I wanted to eat healthy, I had to work hard. Holidays and festivals flowed from one right into the next, all of them centered on food. People travel to NOLA with the sole purpose of eating, so living there meant facing food obstacles at almost every turn and feeling doomed in the process.

As I grew serious about losing weight, I had to evaluate how my social life affected my potential for success. Every interaction with friends revolved around food; my family cooked and shared large meals. How could I plan a social event and not start with the menu? Not until I left home for college did I begin to set the boundaries I needed to manage my weight.

When you feel like healthy changes mean missing out on all the fun, strike a balance by being in touch with your motivations for healthy change and keeping them at the forefront of your mind. When I go into social situations where I may be tempted to overeat, I wear a bracelet that reminds me of my goal. It helps me remember I'm there for friends and family, not food.

Share your goals with friends and encourage them to join you, but be prepared to fly solo if they aren't ready for change. If being around old habits is a slippery slope, look for new ways to socialize. For me, this meant meeting friends for walking dates during lunch instead of dining out, planning active outings, and bringing healthy foods to parties. Eventually, people expected me to cheerfully resist temptation, which is how I earned my nickname: Healthy Heather!

Many times, the people we are closest to help us navigate the ups and downs of weight loss. But those same people may be our biggest obstacles, and we have to consider whether old relationships are compatible with new habits. Friends who sabotage you, undermine your values, or make you feel inferior because you're choosing a different path may feel threatened by the changes you're making and how they'll affect your relationship. Others may be jealous of your success or resentful that they aren't ready to make the same changes. They have the right to feel that way, but they don't have the right to undermine your commitment to change.

When I visit my family in the Big Easy, I still watch what I eat, but I do much better when I stay focused on the real reason for being there. Living healthy when your social life revolves around food can be overwhelming. A combination of preparation, compassion, and downright stubbornness can help you change your lifestyle and still enjoy social gatherings.

While We're on the Subject . . .

Sometimes failure seems inevitable. When every weekend is booked with social events, holidays lurk around each corner, and the cycle of indulging with friends seems endless, you may feel like there's no point in trying. Be realistic. There will never be a perfect time to start taking better care of yourself. Just start. And don't take this the wrong way, but no one is paying nearly as much attention to what you're doing as you may think. Your success is completely within your hands, regardless of the circumstances.

Make Your Own Rules

Surround yourself with people and influences that support the life you want. Seek opportunities to be part of the lifestyle you want to create for yourself. The more you participate in your future, the sooner it becomes the present.

Reflect

1. What aspects of your social life support your healthy goals?
2. How can you foster more of that in your life?
3. Look at your social calendar. What's the first opportunity you can practice your new habits?

WEEK 13

The Rules of Awareness

Many factors have contributed to the complex structures of modern civilization, but I imagine that chief among them is something simple, so simple that we don't even give it a second thought: awareness. Observation. Good old-fashioned knowing stuff. After all, awareness is the first step of every journey, right? We can't make a decision unless we're aware that one is necessary, and we can't carry out plans without awareness of the situation that needs to be resolved. This is great news because this simple, almost automatic response is one of the cornerstones of healthy living.

I say awareness is *almost* automatic because sometimes it's not. We may miss something important and have to retrace our steps. For example, how aware are we of our eating habits, especially during the holidays when, let's just say, nutrition priorities grow a little hazy?

One of the questions folks often ask when they find out I'm a wellness coach is "Are you going to make me write down everything I eat?" The answer is pretty much the same as almost any question related to health: it depends. If one of your goals is related to weight, then you'll want to know about food choices that affect your weight. Food intake is a direct contributor to weight, so collecting information about what impacts your diet makes sense. So, while I won't force you to write down everything you eat, I will recommend that practice and hope you choose to do so, because tracking food intake is the fastest route to change.

But I have some rules—three rules, in fact—that I believe are essential to success when logging food. Don't worry, the rules are simple, and they come from a place of love.

First, if you bite it, you write it. This rule is really "if you swallow it, you write it," but that doesn't rhyme. The goal is to build awareness of how the little bites add up. Once we commit to acknowledging and recording our actions, they're a lot harder to ignore. But this rule isn't intended to be a shaming finger wag, pointing out all the ways you're failing. Instead, consider it an opportunity to step back and take in the full picture of your healthy eating landscape. The next rule makes that a little easier.

The second rule is don't feel bad about anything you wrote down. It is what it is. Tracking food is data collection, not an assessment. Evaluate later what you should do once you've accumulated the data. For now, the goal is collection, not analysis. So, bite it and write it with reckless abandon; be your authentic self all over that food log. You're the only one looking at it anyway, so who cares what it says? You had M&Ms for lunch? It is what it is. Write it down. Let it go.

The third rule is more challenging, like the kid in the back of the class who asks about homework at the end of the day. In this step, review what you wrote down and add a note: why you ate it. Again, this step isn't an evaluation or an assessment; you're collecting more of the necessary information to make a well-informed plan. Be honest about the reason you ate something. Was your stomach hungry? Were you bored, was it mealtime, or did someone bring that food to you? Step back and think about each item, and when that voice in your head tells you the answer, believe it.

That's all you have to do. Eat, write down what you ate, and note why. That's the whole process.

The magic happens on its own. That awareness leads to behavior change in such a powerful way that we almost don't have to do anything other than let it work. If change is a goal, then I dare you to keep a journal of your habits—a true, honest, nonjudgmental, vulnerable account of what happened—and not see a clear path develop before you. Whether you take that path is up to you, but once the path is clear and you're ready to take the first step, you will.

While We're on the Subject . . .

Once we see, we cannot unsee. We can't unknow what we know. Once something becomes apparent, we cannot ignore it or pretend it doesn't exist. That's one of the most powerful, and scariest, elements of practicing awareness. We spend plenty of time hiding from what we don't want to face. And awareness requires a certain amount of bravery—to know fully then decide whether to take action. Be gentle and compassionate with yourself as you discover habits and patterns; you're doing something brave.

Make Your Own Rules

It can be fun to practice observing without evaluating. Give it a try! When new information presents itself, just let it exist a while before you decide how you feel about it. Notice your shoulders relax, your sense of urgency subside, and your breathing become easier. You can observe without an opinion.

Reflect

1. What do you want to learn about your habits and patterns?
2. Close your eyes and visualize your inner self as a child. What does he or she need to hear?
3. If you decided to observe without evaluating, what would you see?

WEEK 14

The Five Stages of Healthy Eating

When I first became serious about healthy eating, I felt overwhelmed. I grew resentful about how much time and energy I invested in choosing groceries. As I mourned my old, comfortable habits, I decided that just as there are five stages of grieving, there are also five stages of healthy eating.

Denial. Many of us think we're already eating healthy food. After all, we buy whole grain bread, Greek yogurt, nuts, and sports bars. But then we learn that bread is full of preservatives, the yogurt is filled with sugar, and our sports bars are candy with a picture of someone exercising on the package. That's when we move into the second stage.

Confusion. We like this food. We feel betrayed when our favorites aren't as healthy as we thought, and we don't want to stop eating them. Why? Processed food taps into the reward center of our brain, and we become addicted to their flavor combinations. Denying ourselves those reward foods is painful, and the grocery store becomes a confusing, frustrating place. That's when we enter stage three.

Anger. As we search for products that don't have artificial sweeteners and dangerous preservatives, we grow angry. Realizing that most of the items on the grocery shelves are laced with junk, we want to sit in the corner and sulk for a while. Life's so unfair. Eating right shouldn't be this hard. Then, slowly, we move toward the fourth stage.

Acceptance. Eventually, we realize that we're surrounded by food manufactured for profit, not health. We accept that change starts with one healthier decision at a time: ours. We take a deep breath and buy some fruit.

And finally, sometimes by surprise, we reach that last stage: **Elation**. We feel good when we eat wholesome food. Really good. We look for opportunities to keep that good feeling going, and healthy living becomes easier. Looking back, we wonder why we waited so long.

While We're on the Subject . . .

Healthy eating is rarely a cold-turkey decision. We evolve into healthier people over time. But that doesn't mean the process is easy. Embrace your position in the process and commit to taking one more step forward on your journey this week. The destination is well worth the effort.

Make Your Own Rules

Start where you feel the most curious and likely to succeed. Most healthier eating is simple, but when you feel like you need expert guidance, reach out to a registered dietician who can provide professional expertise for your unique needs.

Reflect

1. How do you feel when you make a change? Excited? Resentful? Curious?
2. When have you felt the rewards of healthy eating?
3. What is one form of self-care that you treasure?

WEEK 15

Take It Easy for Greater Health

At least once a week, someone tells me about the new challenge he or she is undertaking to lose weight or get healthier—stop eating anything white or cut out all carbs or exercise every single day at their new gym.

One thirty-day "get skinny" online challenge listed about twenty-five no-nos: no sugar, no alcohol, no red meat, no tropical fruits, no fast food, no fried food, and of course, no excuses. Then followed the comments of people who had accepted the challenge and said, "This is what I need to finally get myself in gear!"

I couldn't help but think, in gear for what? Never one to shy away from a challenge, I love and appreciate the thrill that comes from achieving a difficult goal. I get that. Doing the difficult just to say you did it is a legitimate source of confidence and accomplishment. But when the goal is healthier living, success is much more achievable when we make the process easy.

First, let me define what I mean by success. When the goal is to lose weight and get healthier, I declare success when my clients have reached a healthy weight, maintain it through holidays, travel, and tailgate season, and feel confident of their ability to stay healthy physically and emotionally. Most of the time, when people drill down to what they want from their health-related goals, they desire the ability to reach a good place and stay there.

That kind of long-range success doesn't happen in thirty days, and it certainly doesn't happen in state-of-survival conditions. You may feel triumphant and accomplished at the end of your month of denial, but I can almost guarantee that you won't be healthier or at ease with your ability to stay at the weight you've reached.

To succeed and thrive, we need to step out of survival mode and into a safe zone. Ask yourself, "How can I make it easier to do what will lead to weight loss and a healthier body?"

For the sake of simplicity, let's use the most common methods for healthy living as examples: eating healthfully, exercising, managing stress, and getting enough sleep. Instead of asking what should be removed from your diet, ask, "What will make it easier for me to eat healthier this week?"

Instead of signing up for the most rigorous workout in town and jolting your body into boot camp, ask, "What will make it easier to exercise, the kind that gets my heart pumping? What will make it easier to find time for meditation or relaxation? What will make it easier to go to bed earlier?"

Yes, healthy living would be easier if we didn't have to do anything, or if wine didn't have calories, or if we had personal chefs and could quit our jobs so we had complete control of our time. Ha ha. Yes, I know. But in your real life, what realistic steps will make healthier habits easier?

Life is hard enough and presents plenty of opportunities to challenge your body and mind every day. Challenge is good for us, and I love a good kick in the pants to work harder and level up. But if you've been trying to convince yourself that you just need to work harder and try harder to make changes in your health, then I invite you to instead ask, "What will make it easier?"

While We're on the Subject . . .

One family photo album contains a picture of me, about seven or eight years old, standing on the back deck of my grandparents' house, proudly holding a snakeskin. I found that treasure when I took a walk in the woods with my grandmother. My grandparents lived in a suburb of Chicago, so their woods were different from the woods near my Louisiana home, and finding a snakeskin made their woods even more exotic.

My grandmother told me that the snake shed its skin because it had outgrown it and didn't need it anymore. The skin was thin and brittle, and I put it back in the woods so it could decompose, because I didn't trust myself with something so fragile.

Fast-forward to the present day. I'm still finding snakeskins. This time, though, they're old clothes, outgrown toys, and other items that I donate, recycle, or trash. Like a snake, every few months I feel the urge to shed my skin and streamline my patterns, so it feels good to get these physical items out of my house.

The same goes for mental stuff. I value efficiency and work to clear out the physical and mental clutter in my life so I can spend my time in the moment. Do you need to take inventory on which patterns are working well and which ones need to be shed?

Make Your Own Rules

If you want to do some spring-cleaning, some shedding of your old winter skin, here are some ways to begin:

Notice Your Patterns. Sometimes we know which nagging habit needs to be discarded. Other times we're not aware of the ways we clutter our paths until we examine what we're doing. All change begins with awareness, so pay attention to how you navigate your day and allow yourself to discover when something isn't working anymore. This may mean noticing when you're thinking, "I'll do better tomorrow," or "I can't go on like this." Those are signs that you're ready for a change.

It's OK if you don't like what you notice. You're going to change that pattern soon.

Let That Habit Expire. Our habits and behaviors have expiration dates. Do you brush your teeth the same way you did when you were a kid? Do you still stand and talk on a telephone attached to the wall with a cord? No. We change our patterns and habits as the world evolves. When you notice that a pattern isn't working well, it may have reached its expiration date and is ready to be retired.

At times, this process can be difficult because habits and patterns make us feel safe even when they aren't productive. If you find it difficult to let something go, have a mental retirement party for it. Thank it for its years of service, acknowledge the good it did for you, and wish it well.

Welcome the New. The first day without that old skin may make you feel liberated and excited. Other times you feel weird and exposed. That's OK. Weirdness is allowed. Avoid the temptation to go back to your old ways by reminding yourself why you started doing something new.

Reflect

1. If you were a snake, would you shed your skin and start over right now? Why?
2. What would you leave behind?
3. What will make it easier for you to take the first step?

WEEK 16

Dig Deep to Reduce Sugar Dependency

My second son inherited a lot from me. His blue eyes, his love for pajamas, and his hard-headedness are all legitimate hereditary gifts from good ole mom. I also passed down to him one more trait, which he may not consider a gift as he grows older: a sweet tooth.

Last week he wanted orange juice with his dinner, and I told him he could have some after he ate the carrots on his plate. I didn't feel like getting up to pour orange juice, and honestly, I didn't expect him to eat the carrots. But he called my bluff, and a few minutes later interrupted his brother to point out that he'd eaten his carrots and was ready for orange juice.

I was stunned. Despite my credentials as a health professional, I haven't been very successful at getting my children to knowingly eat vegetables. When my son voluntarily ate his carrots, I congratulated myself for being such a good example. Then I was impressed by how quickly he'd responded to the right motivation. But the wellness coach in me couldn't ignore what had been a strong enough motivator for him to eat a vegetable: the reward of sugary-sweet orange juice.

We humans are hardwired to crave sugar; we all have a sweet tooth on some level, and the reward of dessert motivates good behavior at every age. But that natural craving plays an increasingly larger role in the health of our nation as we add more sugar to our everyday foods and consume more calories as a result. For that reason and more, kicking the sugar habit is a common health goal.

But kicking the habit isn't just about sugar. The craving isn't necessarily for sugar but for sweetness. Plenty of foods are sweet without having sugar added, and artificial sweeteners lure us into thinking that we're choosing a healthier option. So, the goal isn't necessarily to avoid sugar but to eliminate the craving for sweets. I know firsthand the discipline required to change taste buds because I've tackled that task myself. It's a high mountain to climb but definitely worth the effort. Here's your guide to kicking the sweet tooth for good, if you want to.

Read the Ingredients, Not the Label

Sugar has many names, and you'll soon discover that almost every packaged food in the grocery store contains some form of it. Corn syrup, cane juice, dextrin, malt, or anything ending in –ose signals added sugar. Take deep breaths as you go through the store to keep your anxiety level down once you see how prevalent added sugar is. We'll take this journey together.

Increase Your Fat Intake

Yes, I said increase your fat intake. Manufacturers add sugar to distract you from what has been taken out: fat. Skip the fat-free yogurt and go for the full-fat version. Stick to the plain variety and add your own fruit—with natural sugars and fiber intact— and some chopped nuts. Or have one tablespoon of peanut butter (no sugar added), which researchers have found will zap cravings quickly by activating hormones that water down your sweet tooth. If having just one tablespoon of peanut butter seems as torturous to you as to me, consider this next suggestion.

Stop Skipping Meals

Now we're talking. Ravenous hunger, when we are most vulnerable to swings in blood sugar and cravings for a quick blast of calories, often occurs when we try to make it to lunch without breakfast or eat a measly lunch and then succumb to afternoon temptations. Stay satisfied and less likely to binge by eating every three to four hours and making that meal or snack a balanced combination of protein, fat, and carbohydrate.

Commit to Quit

Eliminating foods entirely from your diet isn't usually realistic or healthy. If you can enjoy a dessert and then go on with your life, that's wonderful. Moderation will add years of health and contentment to your life. But, for many of us, preoccupation with sugar can hijack an otherwise delightful day and make us miserable. The only way to truly change a habit is to commit yourself to being intentional and deliberate about setting boundaries for yourself and respecting them.

Challenge yourself this week to guide your taste buds toward new flavors and give them time to crave something new.

While We're on the Subject . . .

Sugary foods and addictive drugs share many similarities. Here are some of the most common ones:

1. Sugar and illicit drugs or alcohol are harmful to mental and physical health.
2. Both can cause uncontrollable cravings.
3. Quitting sugar and quitting drugs or alcohol can lead to withdrawal symptoms.

4. Sugar causes the same areas of the brain to illuminate on brain scans as drugs like cocaine.
5. Most people build up a tolerance to sugar in the same way they do to drugs or alcohol.
6. Addictive substances and sugar increase dopamine in the brain.
7. People often binge on sugary foods, such as ice cream, the same way a person addicted to opioids, other types of drugs, or alcohol binges on those substances.

Make Your Own Rules

Anyone who has ever been addicted to drugs or alcohol can attest that they endured more than a few of the experiences on the list above. The same can be said about people who struggle with eating too much sugar. Why? Because both impact the brain's reward system.

The only difference is, except for alcohol, most addictive drugs are either illegal or require a prescription. Sugar is legal, and sugary sweets can be purchased almost anywhere.

Reflect

1. When have you conquered internal challenges?
2. Whose fight over addiction has inspired you?
3. What words of encouragement can you give yourself today?

WEEK 17

Level Down to Healthy Up

On the second day of second grade, my younger son told me from the back seat of the car about his day. He told me whom he played with on the playground, which parts of his lunch he didn't like, and that he asked a friend if he was joining Cub Scouts.

But his friend didn't answer, so he asked again. But this time, he said, he used his level three voice. Teachers may already know this trick, but I learned that, for second graders at least, level one voice is quiet, level two is your inside voice, level three is an outside voice, and level four is a voice you should only use in an emergency. He also demonstrated level five, which you can probably imagine.

Life has volumes, too, doesn't it? The last week of summer break feels like level three (or four) with all the scurrying around and preparation. Then, once children are back in their classrooms, life may feel like level one—nice and quiet, at least for a while.

When I think about these levels, I imagine a volume dial you might see on a radio or an old television set. Click the dial clockwise one notch, and the volume increases. Click it again, louder still. Keep clicking, and eventually someone will holler from another room, "Please turn the volume down!"

In my life, I have a series of dials—one for exercise, one for healthy eating, one for sleep, and one for socializing. I'm constantly adjusting them to regulate the noise in my life.

Imagine being in a classroom of second graders who are all talking at level two. Even if everyone used inside voices, hearing every conversation clearly would be difficult. Some of them would need to dial down their volume.

If all the children spoke at level three, there'd be chaos. The teacher couldn't instruct, and the children couldn't learn until someone stepped in and asked everyone to lower the volume. And by ask, I mean in the way a second-grade teacher would ask—not how I usually ask at my house, which is easily a level four.

Our approach to caring for ourselves has levels as well. At times, I've tried to do everything at level three—100 percent effort on every single task. You can probably guess how that went. Life was way too loud, and while I was busy, not much was done well.

At other times, I worked at level one, and nothing happened. The volume of effort was too low to make any progress.

You see where I'm going with this analogy. Are there areas of your life and well-being that need the volume turned up or down? Which combination is the right level for you to feel your best?

You may be tempted to jump into healthy goals at level three, pursuing all of them with the same effort. Sign up for the new transformative diet program, buy all the special foods, and for a week or two follow the regimen religiously. But then, enthusiasm wanes as you realize you're spending so much time learning a new way of eating and cooking that every other part of your life is drowned out.

You may begin an exercise program at level three, gung ho with new classes and workouts, only to be so exhausted by the end of the first week that you pull into a drive-thru lane for fast food or pick up something convenient to eat instead of cooking a healthy meal at home.

Has that happened to you? It happens to all of us. That's why most New Year's resolutions don't make it to February: we're trying to live life with all our dials turned up too high.

Healthy living is about balance—a balance of effort, pace, and progress. Adjust where necessary this week, and enjoy the hum of a balanced life.

While We're on the Subject . . .

A mantra in my running group is "your race at your pace." You may be tempted to try and keep up with everyone else around you, but you'll wear yourself out and accomplish little. So, remember that this life is your race at your pace.

Make Your Own Rules

At what level are the important areas of your life? What do those dials need to be tuned to this week? The level changes, you know. Sometimes meal planning and nutrition need a lot of your attention—level three. That's a good time to dial back some other areas to a one or two, so you can continue to do your best work.

Reflect

1. Think of the different aspects of your life. At what level are their dials set?
2. What needs to be turned down?
3. What needs to be turned up?

WEEK 18

Stop Stress Eating in Its Tracks

Sitting at my computer, trying to predict the path of Hurricane Irma as it approached my home in the Florida panhandle, my brain wandered to an energy bar in my purse. I wasn't particularly hungry, but I reached in, unwrapped the bar, and ate it. Then, with an unnecessary snack feeling like a rock in my stomach, I regretted my poor choice. Kicking myself, I realized that the bar was a completely mindless, automatic response to stress. Dang it!

Why do we crave sweets when we're stressed out? Under times of duress, cortisol hormone levels are elevated, and our brains know that a shot of sugar is a shortcut to a release of serotonin, which helps us feel happy, calm, and relaxed. Our instinct seeks the quickest path to relief—a sweet treat—and that choice satisfies us for a few moments. But then, as we've all experienced, the relief subsides and the cycle repeats itself.

The uncertainty and confusion about Irma's path caused stress, and as I watched others stock up on hurricane party supplies, I recognized that healthy habits were dead center in the cone of uncertainty for the weekend. And that stressed me out, too, because I care about you and want you to stay healthy even when the weather is weird and we're all on edge.

After my mindless snack, I reminded myself of the differences between emotional and physical hunger. When we're flustered in times of chaos or uncertainty, we often rely on a favorite meal or comfort food to distract us from how we are feeling. But if we're working hard on creating healthy habits, that's a dangerous trap. After all, another stressful situation is just around the corner, and eating our way through stress isn't a sustainable solution.

The good news is you can learn the difference between emotional and physical hunger and stop stress eating in its tracks.

Emotional hunger feels urgent, while physical hunger is more gradual. I suddenly remembered the snack bar in my purse and grabbed it instinctively. With physical hunger, I'd notice I was hungry and be aware that I needed a snack in the near future. With emotional hunger, the need to eat something comes on suddenly and feels urgent.

Emotional hunger is specific, while physical hunger is flexible. I often tell my kids that if they're not hungry for an apple or carrot sticks, they're not hungry. Physical hunger can be satisfied with a variety of options because the goal is to end the hunger not to soothe emotions. If you're craving something specific and can accept no substitutes, you're facing emotional hunger. Find another way to soothe yourself.

Emotional hunger ignores body signals, but physical hunger notices them. All of us struggle with portion size at times, but blowing right past fullness and stuffing ourselves with food is more common when we're eating emotionally. Physical hunger is more likely to recognize and respond to signals that we're no longer hungry and that the meal satisfied us.

Emotional hunger leads to guilt and regret, while physical hunger is feeling-neutral. My mindless snacking annoyed me because the bar wasn't the healthiest choice, and I wasted calories that could've been used later on a healthier choice. Ideally, eating is a feeling-neutral situation. We feel hunger, we eat something wholesome and nourishing, we no longer feel hungry, and we move on with our day.

Skip the shortcut this week and eat to fuel, not feel. Pay attention and avoid that stress-eating trap.

While We're on the Subject . . .

Before you practice this new technique, focus your attention on a keyword I used at the beginning of this chapter: shortcut. Sugar is our brain's shortcut to serotonin, but sugar isn't the only option. Smiles, hugs, kind words, exercise, laughter, and other gestures of love can provide the same payoff as a quick sugar fix. When we eat as an instinctive response to stress, our body and mind are reaching out for comfort and stability. But, as powerful as food is, providing emotional support in uncertain times is beyond its skill set. We have to do that ourselves.

Make Your Own Rules

Pause before you reach for that snack, and gauge your hunger on a scale of one to ten. If you're not hungry, congratulate yourself for stopping, and find a distraction elsewhere.

Eat slowly, pay attention to your satiety level, and remember that you can always have more later when you're hungry again.

Pay attention to how you feel about what you eat. If you don't like what you discover, ask why.

Reflect

1. Most of us spend our lives protecting ourselves from losses that have already happened. What has happened that you don't need protection from anymore?
2. When have you realized that something you thought was going to go badly was going to turn out OK?
3. How instant was your energy shift when you changed your perspective?

WEEK 19

Earn Your Own Trust (Stop Kicking the Dog!)

Do you remember the first time you held out your hand near a dog's nose as a tentative gesture of introducing yourself? Extending your hand signaled the dog that you could be trusted, and the wet sniffing around and possible lick of a drooling tongue was the beginning of a long-term relationship. If you held up your end of the bargain—feeding the dog and keeping it safe and loved—you and your new friend enjoyed a long, happy coexistence together.

But if that dog had been abused or neglected, if it had been ignored and kicked so many times that it learned people weren't trustworthy, you might not have received an affirming nuzzle on your first attempt. You may have had to extend your hand several times, patiently demonstrating that you are kind and trustworthy before the dog believed you could be trusted. Only after consistently proving your steadfastness would you be rewarded with a reciprocal relationship of unconditional love.

Well, hunger is like a dog. When your body signals hunger, and you ignore it, you're kicking that dog. Kick hunger away enough times, and it will simply stop coming around. You may notice that you don't even feel hungry anymore. How do you get that feeling back? What if you want to stop kicking the dog, but he won't trust you enough to come near?

Regardless of whether you hear your body's hunger signals, you still need to eat during the day to fuel your body's energy needs and to manage weight in a healthy, sustainable way. Hunger can show up in ways other than a growling stomach; headaches, weakness, tiredness, grouchiness, and dizziness are all signs that you've kicked the dog. Reconnect with your growling stomach by demonstrating consistently—with regular meals and snacks—that you can be trusted to nourish your body. Feed that dog.

Be intentional about eating something small at regular intervals—every three hours or so—and when you eat, make a note of your hunger level on a scale of one to five, with one being not at all hungry and five being ravenous. Pay attention to whether your hunger varies during the day as you are more intentional about eating. If you're concerned that you may eat too much, pay attention to signals of fullness, such as eating mechanically without enjoying the food or feeling pressure in your stomach. Remember, wellness is about progress, not perfection. You won't master your hunger signals right away, and that's OK. Make notes, adjust, and try again in a little while.

Eating small amounts at regular intervals may mean that at first you eat when you don't feel physical hunger, and that does feel counterproductive. Don't worry. You don't need to sit down to a three-course meal. A piece of fruit with some peanut butter or low-fat cheese, a cup of protein-rich yogurt, or some crackers and hummus are low-calorie snacks that can wake up your metabolism without making you feel stuffed.

As you consistently extend your hand to yourself in a gesture of goodwill and nourishment, you'll be rewarded with that welcome feeling of a growling stomach. That's your metabolism jumping into your lap and giving you a big, wet slobbery kiss like a happy dog whose owner has finally come home.

Once you and your appetite are reunited, all is forgiven. Maintain your new relationship by giving yourself food, love, and compassion. Of course, you'll mess up now and then. That's OK. A happy dog comes home eventually.

While We're on the Subject . . .

I asked my teenager how school was going in his new online classroom. In typical teenage fashion, he provided limited feedback, but in between grumblings and wry observations, he made a comment that caught my attention.

"What was that?" I asked.

"What?" he replied.

"What you just said. You said you try to get back into something-mode. But I missed the first part."

"Oh. Pilot mode. When I get off track or frustrated, I try to get back into pilot mode."

I couldn't suppress my smile, partly because I loved the idea of pilot mode and partly because I was so proud of him for being self-aware and proactive. He then explained that he tries to remember that he's the pilot and needs to stay focused on flying the plane. I asked where he learned such a cool idea and he said, "Nowhere. I just made it up!"

We're surrounded by distractions, frustrations, and unknown elements that provide plenty of reasons for slipping out of the pilot seat and wandering around the aircraft looking for answers, explanations, or signs that life will return to normal soon. We could turn on autopilot for a few minutes and indulge ourselves in that distraction, but before long we need to return to pilot mode and take the controls again.

When we got back home from our walk, I watched him run ahead of me into the house so he could do whatever he had on his mind before signing in to school on Zoom. While we lived under COVID-19 restrictions, I felt like we were flying our family to an unknown destination. But we have a good flight crew, and together we safely landed the plane. And so will you. Stay in pilot mode.

Make Your Own Rules

I also asked my teenager, "How do you get back into pilot mode?"

"I just notice that I'm out of it," he said, "and I remind myself to get back in it."

That kind of nonjudgmental self-awareness is a gentle, compassionate way to care for yourself. In the process of kindly redirecting yourself, you build the necessary confidence to tackle difficult emotions, circumstances, and feelings.

Reflect

1. How do you notice that your body is communicating with you?
2. What signals do you often ignore, even when they persist?
3. How can you respond to them today?

WEEK 20

Rethink That Cheat Day

If you've read to a small child recently, you may be familiar with a certain very hungry caterpillar who ate lots of healthy fruits and vegetables all week long. He was so good!

The weekend then arrives, and our caterpillar friend does what many of us do on the weekend. He goes off the plan. In *The Very Hungry Caterpillar*, he eats through one piece of chocolate cake, one ice cream cone, one pickle, one slice of swiss cheese, one slice of salami, one lollipop, one piece of cherry pie, one sausage, one cupcake, and one slice of watermelon. And that night, he has a stomachache.

The very hungry caterpillar had a cheat day. You know, that one day of the week when you cheat on your diet. You eat whatever you want and throw caution to the wind because you deserve it! You've worked so hard! You've been so good! You deserve . . . to cheat?

A lot of clients tell me stories of being what they consider good during the week and bad on the weekends, adding plenty of justification for having a cheat day. I used to have a cheat day too, and I also anticipated my day off from healthy eating. But over time, I realized that when I set aside my healthy habits, the only one being cheated was me. Food became more central in my life than I wanted it to be. I also recognized that if I felt the need to cheat on myself, maybe I wasn't managing my health in a balanced way, so I started to investigate why I felt the need to rebel.

Rebellion is human. After all, everyone needs a break now and then, and rebellion can be a therapeutic release from the restrictions of polite society. But cheating is different from rebellion. While rebellion comes from a place of confident defiance, we cheat because we don't think we can succeed on our own. Students cheat on a test because they aren't prepared. When people cheat in a relationship, they may doubt that they can bring what needs to be brought to that relationship. When we cheat on our nutrition, we're telling ourselves, "I cannot do this on my own."

You deserve better, and you can treat yourself better by changing one little word. Turn *cheat* into *choice* and step into a positive place where you don't view your health as a test, and you don't need to cheat.

While We're on the Subject . . .

Making the choice to overindulge in food or eat something unhealthful doesn't necessarily mean you're cheating. It means you're human. You have the power and ability to make a healthy choice, but in this instance, you're choosing something else. That's OK. When you're ready to return to your healthy habits, you will. Consider healthy living an open relationship—you're allowed to see other habits.

Make Your Own Rules

There's no benefit in going back over yesterday and what you did or didn't do because you were a different person then. Let go, forgive yourself, seek understanding, and proceed forward, knowing that you'll make more mistakes in the future but can access the tools you need to recover.

Reflect

1. When are you like the hungry caterpillar?
2. What advice would you give the caterpillar?
3. How can you remind yourself this week that you have everything you need to be successful on your own?

WEEK 21

Results Not Typical

"Results not typical." There's a reason for that small-print disclaimer on advertisements for popular weight loss schemes: for every person who experiences lasting success on most commercial weight-loss programs, many more are starting again from scratch. There are plenty of reasons we don't experience long-term satisfaction from these programs, but the before-and-after photos keep inspiring us to see if maybe, this time, we're the one who will strike gold.

In a recent conversation with a client, we talked about the twisty road that leads to permanent health and body transformation. Marketing companies and social media posts want us to believe that a new life is thirty or ninety days away, and they have the photos to prove it. Look at the inches lost and sizes dropped! And then my client made me very proud. She said, "My before-and-after pictures would have to be of my brain."

Oh yeah.

Sometimes you work hard, take two steps forward and one step back, walk the long road to success, and do the inside work for months before anything shows up in the mirror, and you feel like you're not making any progress. But then, you start noticing small changes, like the time you got excited about a bowl of ice cream, and it was just OK. Or one Sunday night you realize that you don't feel sluggish from a weekend of overdoing it. Or you hear yourself order a side salad instead of french fries. Or say,

"Nah, I'm good," to that second beer. Guess what? Those are your before-and-afters.

If you're taking the twisty path, the one that looks more like a roller coaster track than a bridge to change, I challenge you to discover your own before-and-afters this week. Notice when you're doing something different from what you would've done before, and snap a mental picture of it.

When you jog the stretch of road that you used to walk, take a mental picture.

When you pass by the mashed potatoes and get two scoops of broccoli, snap a pic.

When you choose to ignore the voice that nudges you toward the pantry when you're nervous or anxious or feeling antsy . . . remember that.

Keep those mental images with you so when everyone else is showcasing their body before and after their latest diet, you can appreciate the before and after of your life.

Yes, I know you want your body to look better too. We all do! But if you keep making progress along that crazy, crooked path, your results will be visible on the outside too. And when that happens, post a picture for everyone to see so we can all cheer for you. That's hard work, and you deserve appreciation.

But don't discount the before-and-after transformation you can't take a picture of, the one no one else sees. The milestones you reach might not be measured in inches and pounds for a while, and that's OK. When your results are not typical, that's a nice reward too.

While We're on the Subject . . .

When I think of the number of before pictures I've taken, oh my. But you know, as I get older (and wiser?) I find more enjoyment in the daily before-and-afters. What do I mean? Before, I would have written off exercise for the day if my morning workout was rained out. The old me would have assumed that sticking to healthy eating habits on vacation was impossible. Looking back, I see those thoughts as *before* and the way I see life now as *after*. But after what? I'm still the clumsy, hurried, disorganized clod I was before. What changed? Over time, through all those experiences of trying, failing, and trying again, I have somehow developed trust in myself to recover when I get off the track I've chosen to follow. You can too.

Make Your Own Rules

How are your results not typical? Do you see unique rewards for your commitment to living life on your terms? Notice them, then store them in a memory jar or a journal. When following that path gets tough, they'll be a reminder of your unique victories and why the results are important to you.

Reflect

1. What are three small ways your life is better because of a healthy action you've taken?
2. What is one big way you can let go of someone else's expectations of what your results should be?
3. What is one dream you'd like to achieve even if no one else understands why?

WEEK 22

Rest That Willpower Muscle

On Wednesday, things started to fall apart for my friend Amy.

Monday was pretty easy, because her energy was fresh and she was excited about a new fitness plan. Tuesday was smooth too; the novelty of the new routine was still exciting enough to be fun. Wednesday, someone brought doughnuts into the office, but she avoided them, and then her husband surprised her with a dinner date. Mexican, her favorite. That's when the first crack appeared. Unlimited chips and salsa, anyone?

On Thursday morning, she met the day with a renewed focus but a little slower. She found it more difficult to ignore the 3:00 p.m. craving for a sweet snack, and she forgot her lunch. The previous night's leftovers became a dinner she kicked herself for, and by Friday she was wondering why she couldn't seem to get it together. On Saturday morning, she vowed to start again on Monday. For real this time.

I once saw a poster that said, "Exercising for an hour is easy. It's controlling what you eat for the next twenty-three that takes strength." Ain't that the truth. Facing temptation and sticking to a healthy resolve does take strength. I used to think accessing that kind of willpower meant digging in, working hard, and persevering. And it does, but in a different way than I thought.

I have another story for you.

One day I walked with a friend who has been trying to establish some momentum in working her way through a daunting to-do list. She commented that she sometimes rewards herself for accomplishing a big item by getting to relax with an easier task.

Immediately, the analogy to running sprint intervals came to mind, and a light bulb flipped on over my head. Of course! We can make those twenty-three hours easier by strengthening our willpower the same way we become faster on the track: by challenging ourselves with something hard and then giving ourselves a rest with something easier. Not a break. A rest. We may walk or jog slowly, but we don't stop until the job or workout is done. My friend was doing to-do list intervals, which strengthened her ability to tackle big projects without the anxiety that previously prevented her from starting. Brilliant! I did a little happy dance in the street for her.

The key to making it through the week is those intervals. We all need a break now and then; none of us can go at breakneck speed and expect to avoid fatigue. But we can strengthen that willpower muscle by giving it a rest and shaking it out.

While We're on the Subject . . .

Before you run off and grab one of those doughnuts because you need to rest your willpower muscle, let me define what I mean by rest. A rest doesn't mean stopping; it means slowing down. You can rest your willpower muscle by acknowledging that what you're doing is difficult and giving yourself a pat on the back. A walk around the building or the block can let you shake it out and take a rest from being strong. Venting to a friend or journaling your frustrations or tension can give you a space to say, "This is really difficult. I know it's going to get easier, but right now it's hard, and I need someone to appreciate that." And then, you can go back to the heavy lifting.

Make Your Own Rules

We all have limits and can compassionately strengthen them. If you want to strengthen your willpower muscle, pay attention to it. Notice when it starts to get tired, then slow down without stopping, shake it out, and re-engage it when you feel ready to speed up again. Wave to me when you sprint by. I'm cheering for you!

Reflect

1. How do you know when you're living at an unsustainable pace?
2. When have you ignored those signs in the past?
3. How can you notice them now and slow down for a willpower muscle rest?

WEEK 23

Replace "If Only" with "What If"

If only. If only I could get up in the morning. If only I could resist the cheese dip. If only I could leave work earlier. If only I had a more predictable schedule. If only my spouse was more supportive. If only my kids were older. If only my kids were younger.

There is seemingly no end to the scenarios we can imagine that would change everything. When we think about what holds us back, the external circumstances that seem out of our control are to blame. And sometimes circumstances are out of our control, and they do make it difficult to create change. That's OK. Life is allowed to be annoying some days, but that doesn't mean you have to sit around and wait for change. Here are a few ways you can work with the obstacles that try to trip up your healthy strides.

Resistance Is Futile

I saw this wonderful quote in someone's email signature: "Whatever happens in your day, embrace it as if you chose it." We all know that stuff happens, and we can either pitch a fit about it or figure out a way to roll it in with everything else and keep on moving. Cravings will barge into your day, someone will drop a last-minute project on your desk as you're about to leave for the gym, and apathy will wake up as soon as your alarm goes off in the morning. Instead of fighting these visitors, welcome them into the fray. "Hello, cigarette craving. I thought you'd be here today. I'm not doing that right now. Maybe I'll see you later."

What usually happens when we fight the craving for whatever we're trying to resist? It fights back. But when we give it permission to exist without engaging in it, there's no reason to fight it. The craving is there. We see it. That doesn't mean we have to pick it up and carry it around with us all day long. Let those temporary circumstances be. When you stop engaging with them, they'll go away.

Manipulate What You Can and Do the Rest Anyway

Some circumstances, however, aren't optional. We don't always determine school and work schedules. We can't control the weather, the traffic, or the choices other people make. But once we accept them and allow them to be, they can be manipulated or worked around. If the school schedule means you have to wake up early to exercise, well, you'll have a lot of company because many other parents are in the same boat. If the evening commute takes up the time you set aside for a workout, explore opportunities for exercise near your office and drive home when the traffic is lighter. Allowing circumstances to exist doesn't mean letting them stop you. Perhaps you settle for a thirty-minute walk until you can make time for a longer one. Perhaps you set a timer for social media so you can logout with enough time to prep lunch and snacks for the next day. If you want to bring change into your life, you'll find a place for it.

Know What Habits Aren't Worth Changing

A few people I know are rebels. As soon as a routine is established, they are off their schedule after a week or two, doing who knows what because bucking the system is woven into their DNA. Even when they created the system. As a result, they're frustrated with their lack of progress because they're convinced that consistency and sticking-with-it are the keys to better health.

After seeing this pattern a few times, I threw out a crazy suggestion: just go with it. If these people expect to become bored or rebellious, perhaps they should make variety—and the option to change the plan at the last minute—part of the plan. They're happier with a grab bag of options they can choose at their discretion, and their internal need to buck the system is satisfied because they're playing by their own rules. The same can be true for night owls trying to be morning people or procrastinators trying to plan meals a week ahead. The energy we expend trying to change our default settings can be better used when we find a way to work with them. Variety isn't always possible, and results are relative to the consistency of our choices, but if you're OK with that, then go with it!

I leave you with a question to ponder: what would happen if you replaced "if only" with "what if?" What if you embraced that obstacle? What if you just went with it? What if?

While We're on the Subject . . .

A recent conversation with a client was the most fun I've had at work in quite a while. She had set a goal of exercising three to four times a week, which had been challenging because she had a busy job and was exhausted at the end of the day, when she had chosen to workout. But she had lost sixty pounds with nutrition changes and wanted to add in exercise so she could continue to lose weight and tone and strengthen her muscles.

I was a little nervous about her goal because I thought maybe she had bitten off more than she could chew. But a couple of weeks later, she checked in with great success. I asked her what trigger got her off the couch and working out. Her answer was simple and awesome: I love how I feel when I do.

She then told me that even when she had a long day at work and was exhausted, she exercised anyway because she knew she'd feel better right away.

I wanted to make sure I understood what she was saying, so I asked her for confirmation: the results from exercising were immediate, positive, and attainable. Yes, she said. They were.

I was floored. This was fantastic news. Just a few weeks prior, she had been frustrated that her progress had stalled, and she was at a crossroads for what to do next. She was confused, because she was still working hard, but her body wasn't changing as much. She sighed and confessed, "I know, I want instant results. I need to give it time."

But now she was positively giddy, telling me that exercising made her feel so good right away that she was looking forward to her workouts after a long day at work. We laughed and cheered over the phone as we marveled in her discovery. Happiness, relaxation, lower stress—all attainable within minutes and completely in her control. In fact, the two parts of life guaranteed to bring her a lifetime of happiness were two elements she had complete control over: what she ate and whether she exercised. Instant gratification was sitting next to her the whole time.

Make Your Own Rules

Feeling a little low on self-confidence? Battling anxiety? Go and do a strength-training workout or join an exercise class. Exercise can boost self-esteem and improve body image, making you feel like a million bucks. And when you feel good, you look good. More instant benefits. Could this get any better? You betcha.

Not only does exercise immediately make you feel amazing, raise your intellect, and promote healthy eating, it burns calories, which leads to weight loss. Yes! You can lose weight on top of feeling great whenever you want to. Oh, and exercise also lowers your blood pressure, enhances sleep quality, reduces cholesterol . . . should I go on?

Instant benefits are sitting next to you too. You can join my client and feel amazing today. Right now. I hope you will, and that your smile will not be able to get bigger. You deserve to feel great. What are you waiting for?

Reflect

1. What instant benefits are sitting next to you today, waiting to be called into action?
2. What are you waiting for?
3. When have you persevered even though the deck was stacked against you?

WEEK 24

Recalibrate

I traveled to Nashville with some fellow wellness coaches for a training meeting. We had a day to ourselves before our meeting began, so we set out to explore and find food. With little knowledge of the city but a determination to find a healthy brunch in this biscuit and barbecue haven, we turned to our phones for an internet search. And off we went.

We walked a few blocks, joking that none of us follow directions well. We were soon off of our path, but that wasn't a problem. We re-centered ourselves on the map we were following and carried on. We walked and wandered, playing Goldilocks to Nashville's three bears of breakfast options: too crowded, too greasy, too fancy. And each time we lost our way, we laughed and called out that word known by anyone who has relied on GPS navigation and gotten lost: "Recalibrate!"

About the fourth time we recalibrated and three miles into our sojourn for a breakfast that had turned into brunch, I realized that recalibrating is an essential part of any health journey and happens in different ways throughout our lives.

We all get lost on the path to a new and improved us, whatever that may be. Sometimes we make a deliberate pit stop, like deciding to let go of the healthy eating reins during a vacation. Other times the diversion is out of our control, like a health issue. Often, our wandering is due to circumstances we could have planned for but didn't, like transitioning into a new schedule or lack of knowledge about how to take the next steps.

The reason doesn't necessarily matter if we remember that our internal GPS is always there, ready to announce, "Recalibrating."

But for recalibration to be helpful, a few elements need to work together.

A Destination. Your GPS knows you're offtrack because it knows where you're trying to go. Without a clear destination in mind, GPS is useless. Our internal sense of direction is similar. With a general goal of "get healthy," we're doomed to wander aimlessly, lost forever. Once we decide on a destination—maybe not a permanent one, just the first leg of the journey—our internal GPS is a lot more helpful. Decide where you want to end up before you start traveling.

A Connection. If we set our GPS to a destination and then ignore the navigation directions—never looking at the map for context of our whereabouts, not responding to nudges to take the next available U-turn—well, our GPS would be useless again. The relationship between traveler and navigator is fluid. We choose the destination, the GPS suggests the best route, and then we choose whether to take the lead and begin. The map only recalibrates after we start moving. Likewise, we need to be connected to our internal GPS, checking in periodically with ourselves to make sure we're still moving toward our chosen destination.

A Desire to Arrive. My friends and I could've wandered all over and discovered plenty in Nashville that day, but we were driven by our hungry stomachs to focus on our goal of food. We entered our coordinates with a purpose. Reaching health goals requires the same kind of commitment to a purpose and desire to arrive. Achieving goals leaves room for wandering, but the happiest travelers make efficient use of their resources and are eager to arrive at their destination.

In case you're wondering, yes, we found our destination: a shack on the outskirts of downtown called the Blue Sky Café. The food was delicious and healthy. As we sat in the grass and ate our breakfast-turned-brunch-turned-lunch, we realized we had walked four miles. We hadn't taken the most direct route, but the journey had been more fun because we wandered a while. We considered catching an Uber back to the hotel but decided we'd rather walk. After all, the return trip would be shorter: the more we learned our way around Nashville, the less often we needed to recalibrate.

While We're on the Subject . . .

Getting lost is part of the journey. Some people say the best way to learn how to navigate a new environment is to get lost in it. We all need room to wander and explore the landscape of our lives. We may discover that the destination we set for ourselves isn't where we want to go. You can change the destination at any time. This is your journey.

Make Your Own Rules

When I set my alarm at night, I think about how I expect to feel when the alarm rings the next morning and what would be helpful to me at that time. I'm a morning person—usually one of those annoyingly chipper morning people who bounce out of bed hours before dawn ready to tackle the world. But lately, I haven't been sleeping well, and when my alarm rings, my pillows whisper sweet nothings into my ear. So, it's helpful to have thought ahead and programmed my alarm with something compelling to coax me out of bed and into what's good for me.

That's where the option to name my alarm comes in handy. Sometimes I write, "You said you would," if I need extra accountability. Other times I need this reminder: "You're going to feel great!" This week, my alarm says, "It's always worth it!" And you know what? I was right. Give this trick a try when you need a morning boost, and let me know which message motivates you.

Reflect

1. What would your life's GPS say to you today?
2. Choose a destination for this week. Where are you going?
3. How will you know when you get there?

WEEK 25

It's OK to Want to Change

I once posted a meme on my Facebook page featuring everyday women and their bellies—big bellies, flat ones, lumpy ones, and ones covered in childbirth scars. The meme was a beautiful testament to the incredibly impressive piece of artwork that is the human body and a celebration of its strength, function, and value. My friends loved the post. Everyone felt empowered and liberated. We all did a collective fist pump for our freedom to be flabby and congratulated each other for accepting ourselves as we are.

And then, I suspect, some of us said, "But I still want that six-pack." It's OK to admit that you would have been among them. I was.

You know what? You can love yourself and still want to change. Yes, you can. You can think you are great just as you are and still want to change yourself. The key is your reasons for wanting change, accepting where you are now, and connecting with your readiness for the challenge should you choose it.

Sustainable change comes from a motivation that's positive, self-driven, and empowering. Most of us attempt to change a habit multiple times before it sticks. Often, the stickiest attempt is the one that comes from within, not from pleasing others. If you feel pressure to change your body to gain the acceptance or admiration of others, hear this: it's OK to like the way you look even if you're not sure others do. They'll get over it.

Body acceptance is important because one of the first steps in bringing about change in your life is fully accepting and celebrating what your life is like now along with all the choices and circumstances that led to this point. After all, change takes work—maybe more than we're willing or able to invest, even when we have enthusiasm for it. By accepting the past and the present, we can better choose a future.

I'm proud of my body. It's strong and can do some impressive stuff. But it doesn't look the way I thought it would considering how hard I work to maintain it. Despite feeling proud of my strength and endurance, I sometimes hear myself saying, "If only I could get rid of this belly." Does that mean I don't appreciate being strong? Of course not. We're all allowed to want outcomes without making their pursuit a priority. Sure, I could drink less wine and eat less cheese, and I might have better abs as a result. But I'm also OK with that not happening.

It's also OK to want to change. It's not OK to tell yourself that you're worthless unless you do. It's not OK to deprive yourself of love and happiness and compassion because you're imperfect. It's not OK for others to degrade you because of how you are. But if the motivation for change is coming from a place of positive enthusiasm for challenge and the commitment aligns with your priorities, then go for it—on your terms.

Wanting something different while still appreciating what you have is possible. You don't have to choose. If you're going to liberate yourself from anything this year, free yourself from the belief that wanting to change your body or your habits is the same as rejecting yourself. It's not.

Enjoy yourself. You're amazing. Soak in how incredibly well your body has navigated life's ups and downs and appreciate the story behind every lump, line, and bump. And if there's more to your story, turn the page when you feel excited about what may lie ahead.

While We're on the Subject . . .

Sometimes we assume we're being inauthentic if we accept ourselves as we are while not liking some elements of how we are. Today, I suggest that there's no such thing as faking it and that when we go through the motions of pretending to be happy about or competent at doing some things, we're still doing them and therefore not fake.

When you signed up for the 5K race even though you've never done anything like that and say, "I'm going to fake it until I make it," you aren't pretending to prepare for a 5K. You are preparing for it. Real stuff. Not faking.

When you walk into a meeting full of people you don't enjoy, plaster on a smile, and decide to fake it, guess what? Even a fake smile triggers real responses in your body and makes a negative frame of mind harder to maintain. The smile may not be sincere, but it's real. Not faking.

Going through the motions of acceptance triggers actual acceptance by opening your eyes to the possibility that you could be happy in more than one set of circumstances. Go ahead and fake it.

Make Your Own Rules

Practice welcoming awareness. Acceptance starts with awareness—welcoming what we notice without judgment or evaluation. Observe your thoughts for what they are—observations—without assigning an opinion to them.

Try this: close your eyes for a minute, and instead of trying to clear your mind, gently notice your thoughts, feelings, and physical state. All thoughts are welcome, positive and negative. Just let them be.

If this exercise calms you and generates peace, do it more often.

Reflect

1. Who in your life affirms you as you are?
2. Whom do you affirm and celebrate as they are?
3. Do you use the same words with yourself that you use for those you affirm?

WEEK 26

Declare Independence from Negative Self-Talk

The Fourth of July is one of my favorite holidays. I usually spend the day at a big family reunion in Chicago, where my soul comes alive. And I'm a sucker for a revolution. The spirit of independence inspires me, and this holiday is a good time to check in and release myself from bad habits, especially negative self-talk. Let this be the year you declare your independence from the negative self-talk that prevents you from taking your health to the next level.

Not everyone is affected by negative self-talk, but many of us have been at one time or another. Negative self-talk is the voice in your head that casts doubt on, or outright rejects, your thoughts or ideas about what you can do. This whiny voice says, "You can't do that," or "That'll never work," or "Don't even try." Sometimes you can silence it and carry on. Other times, especially when you've had experiences when the voice was right and you did fail, you believe it.

Declaring freedom from this tyranny is easier when you take A.I.M.

A = Awareness. Awareness is always the first step. We cannot change what we're not aware of, so notice when you hear a negative thought. Pay attention when you say something that jabs your confidence. This kind of awareness takes practice at first, but soon you'll be able to identify when you're likely to speak negatively to yourself and stop the voice before it begins. That comes in step two.

I = Identify the source. Once you realize you're speaking negatively to yourself, resist the temptation to push the voice away or ignore it. Stop and listen. Then consider why those thoughts arose. Did you see or hear someone that triggered the negative thought? Noticing what triggers you to think negatively will help you be proactive about avoiding those experiences or being ready with a positive response when you can't avoid them. Once you're aware of the negativity and have identified its cause, change course.

M = Mold. Whenever you hear yourself speaking negatively, mold your words into a positive statement. Be honest and sincere with yourself; don't create a hollow sense of confidence that won't withstand a challenge. Know your strengths and call them into active duty when you need support.

Your brain believes what you say. Declare your independence from the tyranny of negative thoughts and take A.I.M. at a new level of possibility.

While We're on the Subject . . .

Identifying our strengths when we're feeling down is often difficult, but we can always do something positive. "I can't" can be molded into "I have not yet." Do you hear the potential? "That will never work" can mold into "Perhaps if I try it this way." Acknowledge the source of the criticism and then debunk it. If you can't find the silver lining, remind yourself that kindness always wins, and give yourself another chance.

The benefit from all this kindness is that you let go of excuses more easily and embrace the potential for healthy choices even in the face of challenge. Better health isn't an all-or-nothing situation. Holiday weekends, vacations, and unexpected obstacles can make you feel that sustaining healthy habits is nearly impossible, so remember that *impossible* becomes *I'm possible* with a tap of the space bar. Give yourself space to identify when you begin to limit your potential.

Make Your Own Rules

Look at your daily habits and ask yourself, "Are they encouraging me to evolve by taking aim at my goals in life or do they keep me going in circles?"

Reflect

1. Where in your body do you feel tension or release when you notice negative thoughts?
2. Where in your body do you feel tension or release when you identify how those thoughts make you feel?
3. Where in your body do you feel tension or release when you mold a new message?

WEEK 27

Motivation vs. Accountability

Step right up for the greatest show on earth! Watch as two friends become foes when they battle it out in the ring.

In one corner, we have Motivation: a burning, churning force to be reckoned with, not to be underestimated once you grab his tail. But watch out—he's slippery!

And in the other corner, his partner in crime but eventual rival, Accountability. He's always there to put you in your place or tear you down with a trick up his sleeve: the ability to masquerade as his foe.

Who will win when these two forces compete to be the center of your attention? Sit back, ladies and gentlemen, and enjoy the show!

This scene played out in my mind after a conversation with someone who said she wanted me to motivate her to reach her goals. I quickly clarified that she had all the motivation she needed, but it might be lost inside her. My job as a wellness coach is to help folks find their motivation, connect to it, and use it as a tool for success. Accountability is part of that process, but don't be tricked when accountability dresses up like motivation.

Yes, that's right. Sometimes accountability will pretend to be motivation—a sneaky trick used to convince many of us that achieving our goals requires someone else to make sure we did what we said we'd do. The ruse works for a while because accountability adds an element of urgency and excitement—

mostly because we don't want to feel shame or regret when we haven't followed through. But eventually the novelty wears off, and we don't care as much about the approval of others. Then the gig is up. Accountability's true identity is revealed, and we realize that to keep making progress we have to look away from others and toward ourselves.

Motivation and accountability are friends. And accountability can be a form of motivation at the beginning stages of working toward a goal. But we make more progress when these two friends work together.

Are you looking for the right combination of motivation to get going? Ask yourself these two questions.

What? What is it that you need a kick in the pants to do? What outcome do you want? Challenge your first answer with this follow-up question: what does that mean? For example, if your first response was "be healthier," your more thoughtful response might be, "that means I'm not on any medications, I eat lots of vegetables, and I'm exercising four or five times a week."

Why? The answer to this one can go on for hours as we peel back the layers of why something is important and drill down to the core of motivation: desire. Channel your inner toddler and ask yourself why. Imagine this internal dialogue:

> Q: Why do you want to eat more vegetables?
> A: Because I don't want to be on all these medications.
> Q: Why does it matter that you get off the medications?
> A: Because they're expensive and, besides, I don't want to be sick and die young like (insert family member's name) did.
> Q: Why is it so important to live longer?
> A: Because I want to be with my grandchildren, and I want to play with them.
> Q: Why is it important to be active with your grandchildren?

A: Because I don't want to be the grandparent who just sits. I want to take them places and make memories together.

Q: Why is family togetherness so important to you?

A: I want to enjoy my family and be around to see them grow up.

Q: So, if you were eating vegetables and getting healthy enough to get off medications, you'd have more time with your family?

A: Yes. Quit asking me questions. I'm going to the grocery store to buy vegetables.

That is the true identity of your motivation: what you desire in life and why you care enough to do something about it. Putting pictures of your grandchildren on the refrigerator door, visiting them regularly so you remember how you want to feel, and finding friends who share the same goal and support you are all ways to incorporate accountability.

When motivation and accountability step into the ring together, they don't have to compete. They're a great team if we let each of them do what they do best. Let motivation ask the questions that bring you to the exasperated core of what you desire and then seek sources of support that will remind you in a healthy, positive way when life gets tough. Everyone will be a winner.

While We're on the Subject . . .

Once you hit that core motivation—your personal deal breakers, what you are not willing to live without—the rest becomes simpler. Not easier necessarily, but simpler. Connecting to that sense of internal motivation drives you in a different way. That's why I like to say that motivation doesn't ever go away; it just becomes irrelevant. The external motivators that get us going (the bonus at work, the promise of a new pair of jeans, the vacation pictures) are like kindling to the fire. But the internal motivation, what we truly desire and value enough to work for it, is what keeps the flame burning.

Make Your Own Rules

We need a mix of external motivation, like a carrot on a stick, and internal motivation to reach our most satisfying goals. Poke around in your current pile of goals. Are you motivated by a temporary payoff or a personal value? Can you set rewards in place that make you more eager to work hard? The goals with layered motivation will be the easiest to achieve.

Reflect

1. What is most important in your life at this moment?
2. When you were a child, what did you dream about doing with your life?
3. How about now—what is your life's dream?

WEEK 28

Three Things You Have in Common with the Boston Marathon Winner

On what otherwise felt like a regular Monday afternoon, I sat in the glorious Florida sunshine and watched on my laptop as two of my dear friends, and about thirty-five thousand of their comrades, completed the Boston Marathon in cold, freezing rain. Knowing the level of commitment, discipline, and tenacity required to run any marathon, much less qualifying for one of the most prestigious races of our time, I was both awed and inspired. Wow.

Then, I took to social media to share in the energy of the running community, where my friends were posting their reactions to the finish. One post stood out because of the heart icons that surrounded it; a friend had highlighted a part of the race that made me grin from ear to ear. The story she shared is laced with self-doubt, selflessness, and what I hope is a sign of the radicalization of our time.

I didn't think I had much in common with 2018 Boston Marathon winner Desi Linden, but after reading about her experience in the race, I felt a kind of kinship. Do you see yourself in these parts of her experience?

She Had Doubts

It's difficult to imagine that a person who has run all the races required to qualify for the Boston Marathon at such an elite level would ever doubt herself, but Linden admits that in the early stages of the race, she wasn't sure she'd finish. Most marathon runners will tell you that their goal is to finish the race, but we know they have a more specific outcome in mind. So, while her context of finishing a marathon may differ from yours and mine, the concept of self-doubt is universal. We doubt whether we can go to the gym three times a week, or if we can resist the nachos at the ballpark, or if we can keep the weight off once we've lost it. Knowing that an elite athlete I admire has the same doubts I do makes me more willing to keep going.

She Had Help

Desi Linden crossed the finish line alone, but she didn't get there alone. None of us do this amazing stuff on our own. Somewhere along the way, people have helped us, supported us, and given us a leg up so we could gain our footing and carve out a place in the world. We may think we're self-made people, but we're not. Having a strong network of support and guidance isn't reserved for professional athletes or celebrities; everyone deserves and needs this network to achieve greatness. Reaching and sustaining a healthy lifestyle is rarely easy, and we all need help from our friends. If you don't have ready access to people who support and cheer for you, look online at the hundreds of positive communities dedicated to that. Join one. Give the same to others. Ask for help and be the help.

She Had Perspective

This is the part of the story I want to zero in on. You may have heard that during the race, Desi Linden's teammate and fellow runner, Shalane Flanagan, defending champion of the 2017 New York City Marathon, veered off the course about halfway through the race to duck into a porta potty. And in a move fueled both by camaraderie and strategy, Linden waited for her. *She waited for her competitor to rejoin the race.* When they returned to the front of the pack together, Linden eventually pulled ahead and won the race.

So, what does this have to do with healthy living? We all have doubts. We all need help. And even though there's a big skill gap between us and the people who win marathons, there isn't a gap in our ability to persevere, especially when we're willing to slow down and help each other reach the finish line. In an age when competitive advantage and political rivalries dominate the news, sometimes the greatest gains are made when we work together.

While We're on the Subject . . .

Olympic athletes fascinate me. Their gifts, discipline, and work ethic inspire me, and I often go down the rabbit hole of learning all about their training and mental strategies.

Michael Phelps's mental preparation was especially interesting. According to his coach, Phelps worked hard to visualize the perfect race from different perspectives, as if he's sitting in the stands watching it and as if he's in the pool swimming it. He would think through different scenarios and plans for what he'd do if different elements went wrong. And then he would practice the plans so if any of those scenarios unfolds, he was prepared and could quickly adjust his strategy.[3]

Make Your Own Rules

How can we apply that to our everyday lives? How often do we think past Plan A or Plan B to prepare the fail-safe in case we need it? How can you check your safety net to make sure it works?

Reflect

1. What area of your life is calling to you for progress?
2. What would progress look like in that area of your life?
3. What is the first step you need to take to begin making progress?

WEEK 29

Think Wide

When I was a kid, we sang a song in church titled "Deep and Wide." You probably know it too:

> Deep and wide
> Deep and wide
> There's a fountain flowing deep and wide . . .

We sang it with hand motions, and I was a little amused by the lyrics. Did the fountain need to be both deep and wide? I knew the point of the song was that God's love was never-ending, but my rascally brain couldn't help but wonder what if the fountain was just wide? Would we reject it?

The same thought came to mind this week when a friend lamented the recent loss of a job. Evaluating his options, he began to network and schedule meetings with friends in his field of work and hoped that one of them would be fruitful, and soon. A few short-term freelance opportunities looked promising, but he was anxious. "After all," he texted, "I need a full-time job!"

"Negative," I texted back. "You only need to support the life you currently have. You could change your life. Think wide." And the song flowed back into my mind.

We've all had the rug pulled out from under us and immediately gone to work putting life back the way it was. Our lives are deep. We have layers of responsibility, tradition, obligation, relationships, comfort, and safety. We often decide that the life we've created is the only way we want to live, so we insulate ourselves in layers of what we know. We live deep.

But deep can also be dark, and we can plunge into our lives so deeply that we no longer see what's next to us. We're so focused on what's in front of us that we miss opportunities to learn new ways of living and growth.

What if life was wide instead? What if, instead of working to maintain the deepness of our lives, we swam upward and lived shallow?

That sounds bad, doesn't it? Living shallow. Who wants that? You're right. Shallow doesn't work. Let's say, "Living wide." Wide is better.

Living wide means maybe those short-term freelance gigs are rewarding and connect you with new people who hire you for other gigs. Suddenly you're not tied to office hours and can pick up your kids from school.

Living wide might mean that on Monday you go for a walk with friends, on Tuesday you go to the gym, and on Thursday you take a yoga class to break out of your exercise rut of must-burn-calories-for-an-hour.

Living wide might mean you get there when you get there and enjoy the scenery along the way. Wide doesn't mean shallow. It doesn't mean living irresponsibly or without a safety net or a backup plan. It means being able to see the safety net.

What would living wide look like for you? Imagine swimming to the surface and stretching your arms out as wide as you can, stretching your fingers so they seem to be getting longer and longer. Have you been living a deep but narrow life? Is it dark down there?

Come up and look around.

While We're on the Subject . . .

The COVID-19 pandemic pulled the rug out from under a lot of us, making us think creatively about how to maintain our way of life in new circumstances. The deep lives that we had cultivated, including the traditions that had felt so solid and certain, were suddenly sources of confusion and, at times, conflict. We were forced to think differently about how we could create connections, care for others and ourselves, and hold on to the elements that make human life so unique. While the pandemic generated many challenges, we also witnessed some beautiful examples of creativity and innovation. Our lives still run deep, but challenging ourselves to think wide can help us discover new ways to cope with old situations.

Make Your Own Rules

Get your creative juices flowing with these exercises for creative thinking.

Incomplete Figure Test. The incomplete figure test is a drawing exercise in which a scribble on a page is the starting point for, well, wherever you go next. Take a sheet of paper and make a random **shape or** ask someone else to do so. Then, take five minutes to turn the scribble into a picture. Groups can do this too, each person using the same scribble to come up with a different image. Then share to see what everyone came up with.

Thirty Circles. In this exercise, the goal is quantity over quality. On a sheet of paper, draw thirty identical circles. Then take ten minutes to draw something in as many of the circles as you can. When the time's up, reflect on any patterns or themes that emerge.

Reflect

1. When have you had to think wide?
2. How can staying shallow make you think more creatively?
3. What scares you about thinking creatively, and how can you show compassion for yourself?

WEEK 30

Make a Game Plan for Healthy Eating

I've never played a game of football. I've caught a ball of any kind maybe three times in my life, and I used to regularly fake being sick whenever we had to play sports in school. But once a marching band starts warming up and football season begins, something kicks in and I become the MVP.

But we don't have to wait for kickoff to be our own MVP. Anytime is a good time to get your head in the game. No matter what quarter of the year you're in, here's how you can make a game plan.

Prepare Your Offense. Do a gut check on how important the goals you made a few months ago are to you. It's OK to let go of a plan if something that once felt urgent isn't a priority anymore. Think about what does feel urgent and whether you want to pursue it. You have the ball.

Next, plan the offense by determining what needs to happen on a day-to-day or week-to-week basis to have achieved the outcome by the end of the year. For an extra point, take the first step today.

Be Strong on Defense. Even with a smart, solid offense, a strong defense protects that plan. If your goal was easy to achieve, you would have accomplished it by now. But for some reason, you haven't, and you probably can identify the cause because you come face-to-face with it every day. Examine that reason, look for its weaknesses, and tackle them.

To do this, be ready with positive reasons you're making a change and give firm responses to that couch potato in your head. Keep victory in view, and stay excited about how you'll feel when you've created your new habit or reached your milestone.

Be Ready for an Interception. Of course, at times none of that works, and you get intercepted. It happens, even to the pros. When you realize you screwed up, do what any champion does: identify your weakness, patch it up, and get back into the game more alert and aware. Setbacks are inevitable, but winners don't make the same mistakes often.

Celebrate Excessively. I don't care what the referee says, when you're able to make positive changes in your stubborn, overscheduled life, you deserve a victory dance. Celebration is important because living healthfully should be rewarding and fun. The more often you connect healthy living with a sense of achievement and reward, the more likely you'll repeat the process. Give yourself every compliment in the book. Don't hold back. You deserve to feel like an MVP when you push yourself to the next level.

Have I used enough football analogies to make my point? You have every skill and piece of equipment necessary to be a winner, even if you aren't entering the season as an undefeated champion. It's a new season, and all the polls predict you have what it takes to be the MVP.

While We're on the Subject . . .

Winning takes preparation. Have you ever heard that opportunity favors the prepared mind? One of my most successful habits for staying organized and productive is to work from one to-do list and update it at the end of my workday so it's ready for me in the morning. Going to bed knowing what I plan to accomplish the next day allows my brain to rest, and I don't need to figure out the day's schedule when I wake up. Do you have a game plan for your day?

Make Your Own Rules

Prepare Yourself for the Win. Any well-trained athlete knows that mental fitness is as important as physical fitness. Using the power of visualization, resilience, and grit can help us prevent injury, fatigue, and adversity. Think in detail about what success looks like in your life. What habits do you want to consistently practice? What physical changes will have taken place? What needs to be present in or absent from your life for you to feel like you're winning?

Plan, Practice, and Be Ready to Improvise. Athletes practice to the point of exhaustion, creating the muscle memory to automatically perform the rehearsed sequence quickly and efficiently. But even the most prepared football players are intercepted, tackled, and compelled to throw a Hail Mary pass. That happens to us too. Be prepared to succeed, and be ready to improvise on the days when life doesn't go as planned. We've all cheered an unexpected run into the end zone that no one thought would work. That can happen in your life too.

Review, Tweak, and Grow. What has been going well for you? What has been your biggest challenge and how did it go? Are there lessons learned and tweaks to be made? Just as a coach and team view the videotape after a game and make adjustments for the next game, each day is an opportunity to reflect on strengths, weaknesses, opportunities, and challenges.

Reflect

1. When do you feel the most organized and prepared for the day or week ahead?
2. Imagine you decided to change how you organize your time. Which of your strengths would enable you to do that?
3. Who could support you in making this change?

WEEK 31

Lifestyle's New Bad Word

Did you know there's a new bad word? I'll give you a hint: it starts with *sh* but has more than four letters.

The word is *should*. Are you aware that we're supposed to feel bad when we say *should*? It's true! I've read all over the internet and heard in videos about how we should—oops, there I go again—stop being so critical of ourselves and live our dreams. We should also stop focusing on the habits we should avoid, because that's negative, and you can't live a positive life with a negative mindset. Oops! I used *should* twice in that sentence.

When I went to school to learn how to be a wellness coach, I learned a lot of rules for talking to people in productive ways. For example, we're not supposed to tell you what you should do. And we're supposed to notice when you're saying this taboo word so we can reframe your mindset into something more positive and helpful. And yes, I'm telling you our secrets, so if you hire a health coach now, you'll be aware of this coaching strategy.

Should is a bad word because it usually means we're beating ourselves up for making what we consider a bad decision, which leads to feelings of shame and obligation. When we say, "I should order the salad," our brains may continue that sentence with "because I need to lose weight" and then "but I don't want to." Either way, you're doomed to feeling miserable about your choices.

But I don't think *should* is a bad word. We all know what we should and shouldn't do. That's reality. And in my line of work, reality is all we have, so I like to ask people what they know they should do. It's important to know. And that question is the best way to move on to a better question: what do you want to do?

If I confirm what people know they should be doing and then find out what they want to do, we can discover the gap between the knowing and doing, and we can mend it.

Knowing what you should do and aren't likely to do is good, but don't stop there. Explore what you're ready to do instead. What would be a step in the right direction? Do that, and don't worry about whether it's the best solution. Any step forward is better than doing nothing.

While We're on the Subject . . .

Should is a helpful word. When we look around and acknowledge the difference between what we're doing and what we should be doing instead, we can make informed decisions based on facts rather than on feelings of shame or obligation.

Make Your Own Rules

Know Your Needs. Sometimes there's a difference between what we should do and what we need to do. For example, I should clean my baseboards more often, but do I need to? Eventually, yes, but not today. I should get some exercise every day. Do I need to? Absolutely yes. Every aspect of my life is better when I exercise, and my body needs and thrives on it. Exercise needs to be done, and I should do it. You should too.

Know Your Wants. Often, my clients tell me that what they should do is also what they want to do, but they haven't figured out how. I should clean my baseboards more often, but I don't want to. I should exercise every day, and I want to. I always feel better after a workout, and I want that feeling. I should exercise, and I want the feeling I get from exercise, so I do it.

Know Your Readiness. Sometimes what my clients tell me they should do is not what they want to do, but they wish they wanted to because it would be good for them. They aren't ready, or the task is too complicated or too time-consuming. That's cool.

Reflect

1. What do you feel you should be doing with your life?
2. How much do you want to be doing that?
3. What do you want your life's legacy to be?

Forget All or Nothing and Take the First Next Step

Imagine if someone in the lottery office called you and said, "Congratulations! You're one of the jackpot winners. You get to share fifteen million dollars with three other people." Then imagine saying, "Oh, no thanks. I don't want any of the money if I can't have all of it."

Imagine a friend bringing a cake to a party and cutting slices for everyone. She hands one to you and you say, "Nah, if I can't have all the cake, I don't want a slice."

Imagine arriving at the movie theatre and being confused when your friend buys a ticket for only one movie. "What's the point if you don't get to see all the movies?"

These scenarios sound silly, don't they? Of course you'd be thrilled with your share of the jackpot, you'd enjoy a slice of cake, and you'd be content to see one movie. But this kind of all-or-nothing thinking is what we use when we assume we can't begin our health goals until we're ready for everything that entails.

In a conversation this week with a client, we discussed her opportunities to exercise during the week. Like many of us, her schedule is busy, and finding a time of day consistently available for her to exercise was challenging. After a few minutes she said, "Regular exercise is just not in the cards for me right now."

If she couldn't have the best-case scenario, which for her is an hour of uninterrupted time to walk, then exercise was off the table. Not going to happen.

We've all been in this kind of situation. As a chronic procrastinator, I've often been certain that the perfect time to work on a complicated project is after I rearranged the cups in the kitchen cabinet, folded all the laundry, and checked the expiration dates on every item in the pantry. After all, I won't be able to focus on my work until I can give it 100 percent of my attention.

But a portion of the winning lottery ticket is better than nothing. A piece of cake is fine. One movie is exactly what you'd expect. And getting started on a lifestyle change is the hardest part.

In the conversation with my client, I asked, "Which would be better: a week when you walked two or three times or a week when you walked zero times?" She replied as I thought she might: a few walks were better than none. She set a goal to walk at least two times that week, which made her feel a lot better about her chances for exercise.

Which would be better for you this week: one step toward a more balanced, vibrant life or zero steps? Look for opportunities to take one step. You already know about the power of small actions to make big changes. Test the theory.

Make a mental note about the steps you took. Shoot, make a physical note too. Notice the good you're doing for yourself and celebrate how a small healthy step makes you feel better. You may discover more opportunities to squeeze in exercise or make a meal healthier where you previously thought those small steps weren't worth trying.

You're worth the big steps and the small steps. Why wait to feel great? When you start where you are, willing to accept a fraction of what's possible, soon you'll find that you have everything you need.

While We're on the Subject . . .

When the going gets tough, the tough keep going! Oh, that's not how the adage goes? Well, maybe the wording should be changed. After all, those who keep going through adversity make the most progress in their health goals.

Think back to the last time you had balance in your life. A time when you weren't in a hurry, you had plenty of time for your to-do list, no one was depending on you, and nothing unexpected threw a monkey wrench in your day. If this is your life now, congratulations. I want to shake your hand. For many of us, though, competing interests and demands are so common that we sometimes feel as if we'll never sustain a structure and pattern that supports our healthy goals. When that happens, turn to physics to learn how to keep going.

Most of success is momentum: the power and strength that builds in an object as it moves. The longer an object travels without obstruction, the more momentum it builds and the more strength it acquires.

Our habits are the same way. If we allow them to progress unobstructed, they build up so much power and strength that they can withstand even the most chaotic schedule. The key to building this momentum is to prevent small obstacles from hindering our forward progress.

Make Your Own Rules

Show Yourself Some Love. Sometimes the reason we stop is because our inner critic convinces us that we are a failure if we don't achieve perfection or even just what we consider to be our personal potential. I am raising my hand here—this is definitely something I have had to unlearn. Showing compassion to ourselves when we decide to be happy with a portion rather than the whole can be a big step forward.

Aim for Enough. I know how it feels to fall short of the goal and then second-guess everything I should have done differently. To break that habit, consider what you would be happy with. If you don't achieve the entire goal, what would be the first benchmark you'd like to reach in pursuit of it?

Reflect

1. What usually causes you to stop?
2. What can you drop from your to-do list?
3. After you eliminate items from your list, how can you scale what is left to allow momentum to build?

WEEK 33

Keep Calm During Tumultuous Times

One morning last week, as I crawled out of my car in the predawn hours to go for a run with a friend, I noticed more stars in the sky than usual. When my friend trudged up her driveway, also still groggy from sleep, she followed my gaze up to the sky. For a few moments, we stood in awe of the sight above us. A solid five minutes passed before we broke our trance and began running. And the stars followed us.

As we ran, we talked about the stars and the vastness of the universe. We talked about the recent solar eclipse and shared memories of the one we'd witnessed as children. And the stars followed us.

We talked about the news and the conflict between wanting to be informed citizens and wanting to bury our heads in the sand. We talked about our kids' first week of school and their awareness of current events. We each said that a part of our mother's heart hoped our children were blissfully absorbed in their own middle-school worlds and unaware of the tornado of events swirling around them. And, yes, we looked at the stars, and they were still there—silent participants in our conversation.

Life feels big right now. Circumstances may feel so big that the pressure of processing our world is overwhelming. Other times, looking at the stars and thinking about what else is out there helps us remember we're only specks in the universe, a blip on the radar of time. The silent stars gaze down at us as we scurry about, trying to turn this planet into one we can be proud of. The stars have seen that before. We are nothing new.

We live in stressful times, as have many before us. We have an advantage, though, that our ancestors didn't have. We know more about the power of the resilient mind to keep us calm, strong, and present as we tackle some of our culture's biggest issues. Maybe the stars are patiently waiting for us to look up, feel small, and check our egos at the door.

About thirty minutes later, my friend and I arrived back at her driveway. The sun was dimming the brilliance of the stars, and we acknowledged that we'd been lucky to see the most dramatic part of their show. I walked to my car to drive home, and my radio came to life with a news update. I turned it off. I looked up at the sky. I couldn't see the stars anymore, but I knew they were there, watching us. And waiting.

While We're on the Subject . . .

We're not meant to shoulder life's burdens alone. Resilient people know and remember that. Talk with friends who share your viewpoint. Talk with folks who don't. Talk to people about completely different subjects, laugh, and appreciate the lighter side of life. Whether you connect with a friend or a therapist, talking about what you're experiencing is a key step in relieving and moving beyond stress.

Make Your Own Rules

If the daily barrage of current events is taking its toll on you, take advantage of what we know about how to cope:

Take Positive Action. History shows us that resilient people and teams have this in common: they take positive action and become part of the solution to the problems they face. Positive action doesn't have to solve all our problems; it only needs to be a step in the right direction. Stomp around, shake your fists, shout your protest, and then take action to change your corner of the world.

Stay Active and Sleep Well. Even the most powerful, robust machines need maintenance. For our bodies, that maintenance is exercise and sleep. Healthy food helps too. A brisk walk can clear a cluttered mind, and a good sweat-fest can fill you with energy. A good night's sleep gives your body and your busy mind time to recover and embrace another day.

Breathe. When the noise of the world becomes a clashing cymbal, just breathe. Close your eyes, inhale deeply through your nose, hold that moment, and exhale slowly through your mouth. Repeat four or five times, or until you feel calm again. You may want to mentally chant a mantra like "This too shall pass" or "I can handle anything." Both are true.

Reflect

1. How do you express gratitude for your blessings?
2. How do you maintain perspective when life gets difficult?
3. If you could eliminate one part of your life today, what would it be?

WEEK 34

It's OK to Not Be Busy

I apologize if you've sent me an email and I haven't responded yet. Same for voicemail. You see, I'm very busy. I'm important, I'm in demand, and I have so much work to do that I'm sure you understand why you haven't heard from me. But don't worry. As soon as I'm free, you'll be the center of my attention. I can't wait to hear what you have to say. I'm so excited.

That's how I used to live my life, back when I thought being busy meant I was valuable. A long, long time ago in a cubicle far, far away, I learned the snarky way that replying to emails too quickly gave the impression that I didn't have much work to do. And if I didn't have much work to do, then I must not be working. And my job must not be very important if it didn't generate enough work to keep me busy all day. Being busy and therefore inaccessible became a badge of worth. I never let on when my workload became more manageable either. Oh no, I was busy. And I never replied to an email too quickly ever again, lest I be considered dispensable.

I quit that job. But not until after I'd been hospitalized twice for exhaustion and so stressed out that I was sick. The toxic work culture seeped into my personal life, too, and I became disconnected and uncomfortable with the feeling of unproductiveness. Free time felt lazy, and I felt guilty if I wasn't making myself useful. Others have called me an overachiever, but the need to look busy had replaced the sense of accomplishment

I felt when I worked hard to achieve a personal goal. I wasn't productive; I was maintaining an image.

A couple of years ago, though, I became fed up with my lack of courteous communication skills. But setting goals to reply to emails and voicemails within twenty-four hours went unmet, and I continued to procrastinate. Eventually, I connected the dots to that job and realized I had learned my lesson too well, and I was still afraid that not being busy meant I wasn't contributing much.

So I started doing what felt very scary: admitting I had free time. Well, that's not completely true. First, I created free time by deciding to stop doing so much. Slowing down wasn't easy, but the words of that emergency room doctor were still ringing in my ears, and I didn't want to be a hypocrite of a wellness coach teaching others how to live in balance while I was so obviously off the rails. I said a prayer and let go.

Then I had to face the real fear: being OK with not being busy and with not being as busy as other people. I also had to remember that I was still contributing to my family and household and work life even if I was no longer barely keeping life together and too busy to return a phone call.

While We're on the Subject . . .

My poor communication skills were created in a toxic work environment, and until I got out of that situation, I couldn't see the root of my problem. Here are some signals that your work environment is doing more harm than good.

1. You hear yourself saying, "I just do my work and keep my head down."
2. You always feel out of the loop or like there are pieces of conversations you aren't privy to.
3. People stay quiet in meetings, nodding and keeping their ideas to themselves.

4. Cliques rule and gossip is rampant.
5. Creative and innovative thinkers leave because they're frustrated.

Make Your Own Rules

Just as a work environment can be toxic, so can the lifestyle we create for ourselves. Do you have a case of busy-itis? Try this trick: schedule a block of time for doing nothing.

Setting aside time on your calendar intended for reflection or unstructured thought can bridge the gap between needing to feel productive and allowing yourself to rest. If you must be active during that time, spend your time and energy on some of the reflection questions in this book or on a creativity exercise.

As you become more comfortable with the art of doing nothing, you may discover that the practice adds a lot to your life.

Reflect

1. What time of the day is most appealing to you for planning unstructured time?
2. When did you say no to an opportunity or activity and feel good about it?
3. How can you protect your unstructured time so busyness doesn't intrude on it?

WEEK 35

A 9/12 Way of Life

Each September, we pause to reflect on the anniversary of the terrorist attacks on September 11, 2001. As I scrolled through the posts on social media that recounted where people were when they heard the news, how the attacks affected our lives and perspectives, and how we honor those whose lives were lost, one message continued to bubble to the top: America on September 12.

Patriotism was strong, but what resonated the most seemed to be the sense of community that permeated our country. We were united, regardless of the differences between us. But before long, our divisive ways returned, and now our country is more divided than it has been in my lifetime. The pendulum of human nature swings from one extreme to the other, from terrorists trying to kill us to us killing one another.

Events in our personal lives can have a similar effect. As a health coach, I often hear stories of the heart attack that was the wake-up call or the cancer diagnosis that put life in perspective. Like on September 12, these moments of clarity remind us that complicated issues seem less important than the fundamental values of civility and unity.

For some, this shift is permanent, and they live differently. Cardiac patients may adopt a plant-based diet low in cholesterol, take daily walks, and learn how to manage stress to protect their heart. The change requires work, determination, and a learning curve, but the reality check of the alternative makes the adjustments worth the effort, and life is changed for good.

For others, lifestyle change is more tentative, contingent on other criteria. When the day goes well, healthy choices are possible. But if schedules are interrupted or drama erupts in relationships, healthy habits become inconvenient, or the learning curve is too steep. Change is abandoned or considered impossible given the circumstances.

For a while after September 11, Americans were united in our humanity. But as our list of criteria for living in harmony with one another grows, so has the distance between us and our potential. We have more demands. Life must adhere to specific, rigid standards for us to play nice. We say, "no deal," if an obstacle arises.

Can the same be said about how we live our lives and manage our health? Are you one who makes permanent changes, or do new habits last only as long as everything else works out?

Do you live life like September 12, setting aside petty obstacles and striding toward the changes you desire for a more balanced life? Do you look for ways to make the lives of others easier, to smooth their path toward progress as a neighbor? Or do you agree to the plan for change as long as everything meets your requirements?

Reading the accounts of life on September 11 and on September 12, I sensed a shared nostalgia for the day we were united. I encourage you to search for ways to bring a September 12 mentality into your life.

Set your work aside and go for that walk. Life is fast; slow down.

Put on your swimsuit and jump into the pool. Life is fleeting; have fun.

Push that greasy food away, and give your body the good stuff. You're surrounded by people who love you. Stick around for a while.

For a brief time in 2001, our complicated lives were put into perspective, and we held hands in unity. Now we've written a long list of criteria that must be met before we'll consider doing that again.

If you have a list like that in your life, one wake-up call could render it irrelevant. Will you wait for that wake-up call or start living like it's September 12 today?

While We're on the Subject . . .

Once in a while, we come across a book that changes the way we see the world. For me, it's hands down *The Untethered Soul* by Michael Singer. I had to read the book a couple times before I could incorporate the practices I learned, but the changes were profound. Singer teaches us how to use mindfulness to understand levels of consciousness that can enable us all to live fully in the present and let go of thoughts and memories that keep us from living joyfully. In other words, he shows us how to let it go. Once I began to practice the skills he taught, I experienced a transformative sense of liberation. The book was a wake-up call for how much of my energy was consumed by what-ifs and how much energy was available for experiencing life. On some days, I still remind myself to untether, and the practice always feels like a connection.

Make Your Own Rules

Try some of these ways to bring sunshine into someone else's life:

- Pack an extra snack to give away when you see someone in need on the street.
- Clean out a closet and donate items to a local shelter or nonprofit.
- Write a thank-you note or an encouragement note to say, "You're awesome!" Remember how good it felt to get mail as a kid? Grown-ups feel that way about a card too.

- Spend an evening serving meals at a local soup kitchen.
- Pay a compliment to someone when he or she looks especially nice—or even when they don't!

Reflect

1. What does a September 12 state of mind look like for you?
2. What have you been waiting for?
3. How can you use your strengths, gifts, and passions to serve your community?

WEEK 36

Banish the Good and the Bad

Have you been good this weekend? Or were you bad last night and now feel like you should atone for your sins with a diet of water and salad? Before you swear off dessert or slash your calories trying to be good again, maybe the biggest change you need to make is your vocabulary.

Words like *good* and *bad* carry a lot of weight. When we describe our actions as good, we feel great, as if our actions define who we are as people. The opposite is also true: when we make choices we consider bad, our ego takes a hit. But we are not our choices. We are people who make choices, but they don't define who we are. Wonderful people can act foolishly. In fact, most of us are pretty good at that.

I invite you to consider replacing the words *good* and *bad* with new ones: *productive* and *unproductive*. With this simple shift of semantics, suddenly we're transformed into good people making either productive or unproductive choices as we pursue a goal. Ordering dessert for the second time in a week when you're working on a weight loss goal doesn't make you a bad person, but it's unproductive. Skipping your daily walk so you can lounge on the couch doesn't make you bad, but that decision doesn't lead to improved cardiovascular health. Changing your vocabulary will help you see that your worth as a person doesn't change when you make an unproductive choice. You're off the hook. You have permission to be happy and content even if you opt out of making progress.

A compromise is connected to this enlightened way of thinking, though, because the pace of your results is related to the number of productive choices you make. Imagine you're on a road through the middle of a meadow, and it stretches in front of you and behind you as far as you can see. The road is your success zone, and as long as you make productive choices, you'll travel along this path with relative ease. You'll see positive changes in your life and your health because you're living in harmony with your body's needs.

Now imagine that you begin making consistently unproductive choices, the ones you used to refer to as bad. Perhaps your progress has slowed. Your waistband gets tight. You're feeling sluggish and frustrated. You haven't become a bad person, a failure who's incapable of change. No, no, no. You're still the awesome person you were at the start. You've simply made a lateral move to the shoulder with a series of unproductive choices. This scenic pause may have its rewards and could be justified, but while you're immobile on the roadside, your forward progress has stopped. If you're OK with that, stay on the shoulder as long as you'd like. When you're ready to travel forward again, begin making productive choices, and you'll be back on the road to success.

While We're on the Subject . . .

Your worth as a person—your goodness or badness—doesn't change whether you're being productive or unproductive. We may not literally think we're bad people when confiding to a friend that we're going to be bad and break our self-imposed rules. But our brain hears a different message. When you call yourself bad often enough, you begin to believe that you are. You're fine the way you are. Your choices don't define who you are as a person, but the productive ones will get you to your goal faster. If you're stalled out on the shoulder of your personal success zone, that's OK. Your next choice is the first step forward.

Make Your Own Rules

A therapist once told me, "Descriptions are instructions." She meant that the words I use to describe myself or others create a subconscious script for my behavior. If I lament to a friend, "I'm so disorganized," then I'll be disorganized. If I chide my child, "You worry too much," then I shouldn't be surprised when my kid sees himself as a worrier.

This week, pay attention to the words you use to describe yourself, either internally or out loud. Are you creating a script for a show that you want to watch?

Reflect

1. What productive choices would move you toward the life you want to live this week?
2. What actions would be unproductive?
3. Which productive choice are you the most excited about today?

WEEK 37

Do You Eat to Live or Live to Eat?

A friend recently sighed, took a sip of coffee, and said, "I envy people who can eat to live, not live to eat. I wish I could learn to do that." I completely understood. For a long time, I lived to eat. I grew up in a culture where gathering around food and cooking our favorites was a family pastime, but over time, I became frustrated with the value I placed on food. Like my friend, I wanted to learn how to eat to live, not be preoccupied with what I was going to eat next.

Health and fitness guru Jack LaLanne is credited with coining the phrase, "Eat to live, don't live to eat," meaning that we should eat with function and purpose in mind, not with enthusiasm and anticipation of flavors and textures that we enjoy.[4]

Do you eat to live or live to eat? Here's a quick quiz to help you figure it out.

When you are hungry, do you (a) choose a food that's convenient and satisfying or (b) reach for your favorite snack, which you've been looking forward to all morning.

When you discover that your preferred food isn't available, do you (a) eat something else and move on or (b) feel annoyed, as if you've been cheated out of an experience.

When you choose a food to eat, is it (a) because your stomach is growling or you recognize some other sign that your body needs food or (b) because it's time to eat or because you planned to eat at that time.

In social situations, do you find that you're (a) looking forward to the food that will be served and anticipating sharing the food with your friends or (b) looking forward to the people who'll be there and knowing you'll eat too.

If you chose mostly As, then you're likely eating to live. That means that while you may enjoy your meals, it's also OK if your food is less than ideal because its purpose is to satisfy hunger, not your taste buds.

If you chose mostly Bs, you may feel that you live to eat. Food may play a central role in your life and be the byproduct or the motivation for your social activities.

Neither mindset is inherently good or bad, and you may land somewhere in the middle. Enjoying and savoring food is a beautiful part of a rich, fulfilling life. Delicious food is part of what makes life fun and brings people together. I'm in favor of tasty food.

On the other hand, some people want to sever their emotional tie to food and join the other camp: people who eat to live. While many may consider this relatively Spartan existence to be missing the spice of life, others may see this as a way to change emotional or disordered eating patterns. Or they may not be interested in food, and that's OK too.

As I say about most habits, it's not a problem unless it's a problem.

Since most of us want to learn how to eat less emotionally, here are some ways you can raise your awareness of your eating habits and learn how to eat to live. (You may want to learn to enjoy and savor your meals rather than going about them methodically, but I don't know many people who are striving for that goal.)

First, notice how you feel when you're around food. What's the ratio of socializing to eating when you're with friends? How do you feel when eating during social events is delayed or not included? Consider whether you're placing too much emphasis on the role of food in your social life and try to focus on friends, fun, and fellowship before food.

Next, pay attention to your motivation for eating. Are you choosing foods you feel you deserve or have earned? Make an intentional choice to wait until you're hungry, and then pay attention to what drives your choice of food.

Finally, try to separate how you feel about food and what food needs to do. That doesn't mean you always pick the productive choice, but be aware of what you're choosing, how often, and how much sense that selection makes given your hunger level and goals.

How did eating get so complicated? I hope you enjoy every meal this week, whether you're savoring the flavors or the efficiency.

While We're on the Subject . . .

Have you ever said that you're ready, willing, and able to tackle the task at hand? The phrase rattles off the tongue effortlessly, conjuring images of a soldier in uniform stepping up to the front lines with a salute, ready for battle. I've said it often without a second thought, but recently I wondered if perhaps the order should be changed to able, willing, and ready.

The beauty of working toward change is that it's a fluid process. Rarely do we get up, begin acting differently, and never look back or veer offtrack. So, if the speed at which you're trying to change is too fast, slow down. You can even go back to the old way. It's your choice.

My question for you this week is, are you able? Yes. Are you willing? Perhaps. Are you ready? Well, ready or not, your life is here. Jump on in.

Make Your Own Rules

Able. This first stage is easier, because most of our healthy living goals involve tasks we can do. With a few exceptions, we can buy fruits and vegetables instead of cookies and soda at the store, drive to the gym for an exercise class or walk in the neighborhood, and turn off the lights and go to bed at a certain time. Our arms and legs enable us to do those things, and we're adults, so generally we have some level of control over our time. For some of us, these behaviors are a challenge, but on average, our functional ability is high; we're able to do most anything.

Willing. Now we move into rougher terrain. After all, what we're able to do and what we're willing to do can be quite different. Sure, you're able to get in the car and drive to the exercise class, but are you willing to miss something else to do that? You have the ability to sip coffee or tea while others have dessert, but are you willing to? You may need some time to sort out what you're willing to do, and miss out on, to achieve a particular outcome. Be honest with yourself about what level of hassle you're willing to tolerate so you can progress toward a goal that's important to you.

Ready. This is where we get to the good stuff. Being able to do things is a gimme, and being willing to do them feels like we're being talked into something. But ready? That's exciting! Being ready to take action is a great place to be because that's where you are: ready for something. The best way to figure out your level of readiness is to think about what feels like a step in the right direction without being too much work. For example, you know you're able to buy fruits and veggies for snacks during the week, and you might agree that you're even willing to eat fruits and veggies as snacks a few times a week. The next step is determining what you feel ready to do. Maybe you feel ready to bring them to work so they're available when you need a snack.

Reflect

1. What are you able to do for your well-being?
2. What are you willing to do to take care of yourself?
3. What are you ready to do today?

WEEK 38

Seeing Fitness Is Not Always Believing

How often do you roll your eyes at an impossibly fit friend who still thinks she is fat? "Look in the mirror!" you may exclaim in exasperation, "You look great!" Chances are she's not fishing for compliments. While some people suffer from the serious mental condition known as body dysmorphia, many of us merely have inaccurate impressions of our bodies that prevent us from appreciating the wonderful ways we take care of our health.

When do we make the transition from a happy-go-lucky child jumping into a swimming pool to a self-deprecating adult who can't see beyond the size of our jeans? Years of yo-yo dieting, social pressure to reach an unrealistic ideal, and letting media images influence what we think our bodies should look like take a toll on us. The airbrushed pictures of male and female celebrities we see in the grocery store checkout line become a basis for comparing our bodies to our expectations or our perception of how we measure up to the expectations of others. But those magazine covers don't have to be our judge and jury. Here's how you can check yourself before you wreck yourself and see the beauty everyone tells you is there.

Before consulting the scale for your daily validation of self-worth, consider what your body can do. And if you aren't sure, test it! A body that can withstand a challenging fitness class, a running workout, a hike in the woods, or other endurance activities isn't unfit. Assign some numbers to what you do to support your own health: miles walked, weight lifted, minutes spent in your target heart-rate zone for building cardiovascular health. These are the numbers that matter.

If you aren't happy with what your body can do, start making it more impressive. Healthy living is in the doing, not the having. Do what defines fitness for you, and your body will get with the program.

Before asking a magazine to tell you whether you're too skinny or too fat, look in your closet. Has there been a dramatic change in the way your clothes fit over the past year? Are you physically comfortable in your clothes when you aren't looking in the mirror? If obesity is an issue for you, take the steps necessary to bring yourself into a healthier place. Take pictures along the way to see your progress over time, preferably of you being active, and look at them when you need a reminder of how far you've come.

Surround yourself with proof of your healthy habits. If you participate in local 5K races, tack your race bibs to a bulletin board where you can see them. If you pride yourself on healthy cooking, display your cookbooks in a place where they remind you of that priority. Keep a chart of how many miles you've walked or run over the course of the year on your pantry door as a reminder that living fit is what you do, no matter what you look like.

And finally, listen to yourself. Our brains believe what we tell them, and negative self-talk can have a permanent impact. If you hear yourself saying, "I'm so (fill in negative adjective here)," stop and replace it with a positive statement that has nothing to do with you: "I'm so happy the sun is shining today," "I'm so lucky to have so many great friends," or "I'm so thankful for coffee."

Here's the good news: you don't have to look like any of those people in magazines. You can look like you and still do everything you want to. Healthy living has no dress code. Do what defines fitness for you, and your brain will start to see your beauty.

While We're on the Subject . . .

Have you ever received directions from someone who includes signals that you messed up and need to correct the course?

> "If you see the red barn, you went too far."
> "If your soup is too salty, add a potato."
> "It's all fun and games until your jeans don't fit."

Life is a constant cycle of learning and, if we're smart, adjusting our behavior as we do. I often encourage my clients to "do the best you can until you know better and then do better." But this week I wondered how often we pay attention to the signs that we're doing well instead of looking for signals that we're not.

My light-bulb moment came in a conversation with someone who enjoys endurance running but has a habit of being so enthusiastic that she overtrains and either gets injured or experiences burnout. We discussed her life as a pendulum swinging from one extreme to the other, and she said she wants to keep her pendulum closer to the center.

As we discussed how she could do that, I asked how she knows her pendulum is swinging too much. "I don't sleep well even when I'm tired," she replied. "I don't look forward to my runs, and I wake up starving in the morning like I didn't eat enough the night before."

Then we switched gears, and I asked the other side of the question: how do you know when you are doing things well? That was trickier for her to answer. The signs that life is in balance are quiet, calm, and subtle, so we don't notice them as much as the loud, frantic, obvious signs of imbalance.

Make Your Own Rules

You can rewrite those pieces of advice so they're proactive instead of reactive: "If you see the red barn, slow down. You'll turn left soon."

Staying on track with health goals requires a bit of multitasking. You need to know where you're going, where you are, and what's coming up so you don't miss your turn.

Apply this to your life by knowing what daily activities ensure that you're thriving. One client knows she's on her healthy path when she does at least fifteen minutes of yoga or walking each day and drinks her water. The first sign of progress is that you haven't made a U-turn in a long time.

"Follow the recipe, and season to taste." Popular culture would have us believe otherwise, but there's nothing new to healthy living. Eat lots of vegetables, drink water, exercise daily, and chill out. That's the recipe to healthy, balanced living, and we only get messed up when we think we know better and start adding our own ingredients.

The second sign of progress is that results are predictable if we follow life's recipe and season to taste rather than improvising and then correcting it later. For my clients, that often means reducing the medications they take or avoiding new ones because their lifestyle has improved. What a satisfying signal of progress.

Reflect

1. What signals indicate that you're doing well?
2. What signposts would you put along your life's road?
3. What visual reminder can reflect your progress and accomplishments this week?

WEEK 39

Bump into the Walls of Your Goals

Imagine that you've moved into a new house. You've done that before, right? Do you remember how it felt to be unsure which switches turned on certain lights or to wake up at night and wonder how to get to the bathroom?

Adjusting to a new location takes a while. You learn how to fold the towels so they fit in the linen closet. You figure out how long it takes the water to warm up in the shower and which room is the coldest at night. But you have to live there for a while before the house feels like home.

Now imagine that you've been in your new place for a few days. While you're still unpacking and surrounded by boxes, someone barges in and says, "Tell me where the can opener is!"

Startled, you may look around at the half-unpacked boxes scattered about and stammer, "I'm not sure."

"Oh really," says the intruder, crossing his arms with a self-satisfied smirk. "You've been here a full week and don't know where the can opener is? I'll bet you'll never know. This whole idea was stupid. This house will never work!"

You may get defensive. "Well, hang on a minute, mister. I just got here, and I haven't unpacked. Give me a few days to get organized, and then I can tell you where the can opener is."

He may shrug, turn on his heel, and sit in the corner, waiting to be proved correct.

That conversation sequence may seem ridiculous, but similar health scenarios happen more than we think. How many times have you been on a diet for a week and then stepped on the scale only to see little to no change? The voice that says, "I told you so," is the same one who barges in and demands the can opener. But when the conversation happens on the scale, we don't get defensive and stand up for ourselves. We hang our heads and say, "You're right. This was dumb. This'll never work."

In your new house, you did find the can opener. You figured out the light switches. You learned how to jiggle the door so the deadbolt will lock. And now, after living there awhile, you can find your way around in the dark. You know which part of the floor squeaks and where to watch for LEGO blocks. You know that place like the back of your hand because you stuck around long enough to unpack the boxes and figure out the new layout.

The same is true with the habits that we cultivate. We've barely begun, but we're demanding results and expecting to be proficient in our new skills. If we don't lose weight fast enough, or we overeat during a weekend of travel, or nothing happens for a while, we assume change will never happen. But it's OK to bump into a few walls while you're finding your way around a new health plan.

This week, give yourself time to bump into the walls and try a few light switches before you call it quits on your health goals. Give yourself some space to learn. Keep unpacking.

While We're on the Subject . . .

One of the most difficult parts of my job as a health coach is being patient when I can see the potential for someone to make radical changes in their lifestyle, but he or she isn't ready for them. At times, it seems to take forever for the pieces to come together, but I know from experience that we can't rush the adjustments. I also know how to listen for clues that change is near.

You See Your Goal Everywhere. Kind of like when you're pregnant and you see other pregnant women, or you buy a new car and see other people driving the same car around town, your goal will show up all over the place. You may notice people walking for exercise in your neighborhood or find yourself drawn to the grocery store's produce section. I don't have scientific evidence for why this happens, but it does. Pay attention and go along with it! When your goal lies down in front of you, stop and pick it up.

The Thrill Is Gone. When I travel, I like to sample local beer and look for restaurants that serve beer we don't usually get in Tallahassee. The splurge of having a delicious, thick stout with my meals feels decadent and special. But after a few days of that much beer, the magic disappears. When I get home and beer finds its way to me, I'm tired of it. That's another clue. When what used to be a fun diversion has become par for the course, it's time for a change. Stop pressing Repeat on a habit that's run its course. Take the hint and change directions.

The First Step Feels Like a No-Brainer. This is where it gets personal: the first step. Some folks would have us believe that the first step is doing something dramatic such as eliminating a food group or signing up for a big challenge at the gym. For some, those steps feel right. For others, they're overwhelming and discouraging. Pay attention to how you feel and move toward what feels like the first step in the right direction, even if that step seems small. When you're choosing between a cheeseburger or a salad for lunch, choose the salad. When you're choosing between a salad with cheese or one without cheese, choose the one without. When you're choosing between a dessert of brownies and ice cream and one of sorbet with fresh fruit, choose the fruit. Notice that I didn't say the step would be easy. It may not be. But it will feel obvious. It's obvious for a reason.

Make Your Own Rules

If bumping into the walls of your goals seems easier said than done, share some of these mantras with that intruder:

"I'm Learning." Yes, there's a learning curve to creating health habits. Remind yourself that you're learning and give yourself credit for what you've figured out. You can even keep a notebook of your discoveries as a visual reminder of what you've learned.

"Give Me Some Space." I don't know about you, but I find it almost impossible to work when someone is reading over my shoulder. My fingers get wonky, and I can't type; I make careless mistakes and get aggravated. I need some space. You might too. This mantra may work best when you physically stretch your arms out to the sides and literally make some more space for yourself. This is your goal, and you can take up all the room.

"Keep Unpacking." A picture on the wall of my living room is crooked—and has been for about four years, ever since I hung it up. Once in a while, I note the crookedness and admit I should take the nails out and straighten the picture. But I haven't. That's OK. It reminds me that I'm a work in progress, always settling in. Allow yourself to keep unpacking and get settled before you decide the place doesn't work for you.

Reflect

1. When have you been patient with yourself as you learn something new?
2. What encouragement do you give to friends who try something new?
3. What mantra can you use this week to remind yourself to be patient when you're learning new things?

WEEK 40

Make Eye Contact with Your Scary Goals

A few years ago, when grocery store shelves were stocked with Halloween candy and holiday sweets, I brainstormed with a client on how to avoid sneaking into and out of the growing supply of Halloween candy in her pantry. I noticed we were making what I call Band-Aid goals. Band-Aid goals are quick solutions; they stop the bleeding and sometimes solve the problem, but other times they only cover up what needs attention. Eventually, Band-Aid goals fail because they don't address the injury. They cover up the ugly wound we hope will heal itself.

In my client's situation, the Band-Aid goal was buying candy she didn't like, asking her husband to hide it, or putting it out of sight so she'd be less tempted to eat it. These action steps were a good start. They took care of the immediate issue—ready access to tempting candy—and could help her manage the Halloween season.

But what happens after Halloween? What happens when the pies, cookies, and special foods come out at Thanksgiving? What happens when you have a holiday party every weekend? That Band-Aid may lose some of its stickiness.

Today, friends, we're ripping off that Band-Aid and looking at the ugly mess underneath. We're making eye contact with those scary goals. Don't worry, you're ready for this, and it won't be that scary. Looking at the scary goals means reflecting on what you're so afraid of in the first place.

After all, what would happen if you did eat all the candy? Why do you need to hide the bags? The answers are a combination of practical reality and introspective feel-good stuff. The practical reality is that you'd probably ingest too many calories, gain weight, and feel sick. That's not helpful. The introspective feel-good stuff is that you might feel defeated, discouraged, and negative about your ability to exercise self-control. Ain't nobody got time for that, so we hide away the stuff that makes us feel vulnerable so we don't have to see it.

Face your fears, make a plan, and be honest with yourself. Rip off the Band-Aid! The wound might look ugly, but it's a lot less scary when you're armed with the reasons a different choice is important.

While We're on the Subject . . .

I spend a lot of time talking with people about their health, and at least once a week someone asks my opinion on the latest supplement, surgery, workout, or cleanse. My answer is almost always the same: there's no magic pill; there's only magic you.

Medical aids can help you lose weight, but they don't change your habits. Embracing a new workout fad can help you break through a plateau, but it won't last forever. Doing a cleanse may make you feel like you're cleaning toxins from your body and refreshing your immune system. If you enjoy that, then go for it. But please know this: no magical power in any of those aids will change your life permanently. The only power that exists to change your life is the power that resides in you.

Diet pills can help you eat less, but you're the one who eats less. Workouts can help you burn fat, but you're the one who does the workout. Cleanses can help you feel lighter, but you're the one who decides how you feel. The common denominator is you and what you decide to do. When the pills run out, the workout is done, and the cleanse is over, you're left with yourself. You keep the ball rolling. You.

Are you feeling overwhelmed? Don't give up. The magic is in your hands, which means you control how much gets changed and when. Even better, you get all the credit. The sense of satisfaction and the ownership of that achievement will be so much stronger when it comes from your positive, proactive actions rather than a shortcut that gives a quick but inflated sense of success that is short-lived.

This week, slow down and ignore the temptation to buy a magic shortcut to what feels like the finish line. Challenge yourself to identify what you're hoping to avoid by opting for that shortcut. Then put your money back in your pocket, take a deep breath, and look inside yourself, where the real magic is.

Make Your Own Rules

Hiding the candy, using smaller plates, holding a water bottle, staying away from the buffet table, and repeating a mantra are effective action steps that work during a single event to get you to the next safe place. Keep using those techniques. But if you need to pull them out every weekend, make eye contact with what you're trying to avoid by asking these questions.

- What would happen if . . .?
- Am I OK with that?
- If not, why?
- Why does that matter to me right now?

Be honest! What would happen if you gave in to the urge? Are you OK with that? You might be, and that's OK to know. But you might not be happy with that choice, and if you're not, then explore why you'd be unhappy. What does that choice represent to you? Why is it a deal breaker? Why is that outcome unacceptable to you? Listen to yourself, believe what you hear, forgive whoever played a role in you feeling that way, and promise to be a better advocate for your real needs.

Reflect

1. What would happen if you were unleashed from the rules? What would you do first?
2. Think back to a time when you felt liberated and free. What made that happen?
3. What would ripping off the Band-Aid mean to you?

WEEK 41

Get What You Need

Sometimes the universe sends us messages.

As I drove through town, minding my own business and going about my errands, the lyrics from "You Can't Always Get What You Want" by the Rolling Stones got my attention. They reminded me that while I can't always get what I want, I can get what I need.

That's ironic, I thought. I'd been thinking about what I want, the unfairness of life, and the injustice I suffer when I can't have what I want. But that's how life goes sometimes. The going gets tough, and the tough keep going even when life's not fair. After all, those who persevere through adversity make the most progress in their health goals. If they keep rolling, they can get what they need.

The key to keeping them rolling is preventing small obstacles—what we want but don't need—from hindering our forward progress. But in this hectic world, these distractions pop up every day and try to thwart our healthy habits. When you wonder if you'll ever generate enough momentum to achieve what you want, take time to stop, drop, and roll.

Stop. When competing interests head for battle, stop and assess the situation. On some days, whatever is threatening your workout or healthy eating plans is urgent and needs attention. Other times, the circumstance seems urgent because it's unexpected. Recognize when this happens and how often you find yourself being interrupted. Why is that happening? Is your day structured in such a way that it's open to negotiation? And most importantly, can you deal with the unexpected situation while still maintaining forward progress in your health goals? Most of the time, there's a way.

Drop. Look at your to-do list for the day and determine if anything can be rescheduled, mitigated, or eliminated. Let's be honest: is there ever an end to your mental to-do list? We'll never complete everything we could do. But there is an end to what needs to be done each day. Some things on that list could wait a day without creating chaos. Choose what's least likely to cause a revolt and shift it to another day. That will allow you to keep moving and build momentum on the habits that best support your life's vision.

Roll. Just roll with it. Crazy stuff is going to happen. Can you recall a day when everything went your way? Exactly. Laugh, shrug it off, and find a way to keep rolling. The key in this step is keeping the goal manageable enough to roll even when you're dodging obstacles from all sides. When you have a lot of people to care for and an unpredictable work schedule, training for a marathon is a big ball to roll. But a morning jog or walk can be managed. Set a goal that can roll. The longer it rolls, the stronger and more powerful it becomes.

We don't always get what we want, but we can give ourselves what we need when we rely on the momentum of one success after another. Look at the road ahead, clear the path, and keep on rolling.

While We're on the Subject . . .

We all know Aesop's fable about the hare and the tortoise. One was fast but overconfident and undisciplined. The other was slow but methodical, focused, and consistent. And we know who won the race and why.

The first step is usually the hardest, but the second or third may be more important. Repetition creates momentum, and I recommend repeating your new habit as often as possible right out of the gate. Do it every day. You don't have to invest a lot of time in it but keep it rolling as often and consistently as possible.

Make Your Own Rules

Building momentum with habits gets easier when we bundle them, letting the success of one new trick be the foundation for the next one. Once a morning walk is established and rolling, it's easier to increase the intensity or duration or to add some stretching before or after. Let one habit get going before you add a new one. Then keep adding habits until you've created the life you want.

Reflect

1. What can you stop doing to lighten your load for the goals that matter?
2. How can you structure your goals so you can repeat them consistently?
3. Where can you see momentum taking you?

WEEK 42

Enjoy Celebrations without Food

For a friend of mine, Valentine's Day was the perfect storm. On top of the already tempting abundance of chocolate gifted to her, February 14 was her daughter's birthday. There was cake. Chocolate cake. Chocolate cake baked by her other daughter.

Before 8:30 a.m., she told me, "I already blew it. I had cake for breakfast." Then she dug down to the root of her dilemma: "How do we get away from justifying bad food choices with special-occasion thinking?"

I'll answer that question by using a few examples that don't seem to be related but will eventually merge into a valid point. Here we go.

Mel Brooks produced and directed *Robin Hood: Men in Tights*, which I love because it's silly and always makes me laugh. In the film, Rabbi Tuckman, a parody of Friar Tuck, justifies drinking the sacramental wine that he carries by blessing everything around him. He blesses the trees, the birds, the squirrels, and the air. The scene reminds me that there's always something to celebrate. We can make any day a special occasion.

Growing up in Louisiana, we had a lot to celebrate. New Year's rolled right into Mardi Gras, and then it was crawfish and festival season. Spring brought a series of family birthdays, which went hand in hand with summer vacations when we, of course, celebrated something else. Football season arrived in August, followed by Halloween. Once Halloween hit, you might as well put on the stretchy pants for Thanksgiving and Christmas. For those of us who vowed to start our diets after the holiday, well, that day never came.

In 2011, I swore off sweets once and for all. That's right, I haven't had dessert since. People often ask, "Not even on your birthday? How will you celebrate your birthday if you don't have cake?" With a party, of course. Who needs cake when you're surrounded by the sweetest people in the world?

One of the biggest hurdles my clients face every day in their pursuit of better health is the office break room followed by the monthly office birthday celebration. Cake! Everyone comes downstairs and eats cake together. And that's cool. Cake is delicious.

At one event, someone asked me, "What do you suggest instead of cake at the office birthday celebration?" How about everyone says something they appreciate about the person being celebrated? How about a fun game to build camaraderie and be silly at work in celebration of someone on the team? And then if you want to eat cake because it's someone's birthday, go ahead. But every day is someone's birthday. That's a lot of cake.

Here's the point. There's a reason to celebrate every day, and if you want to, you can justify eating cake for any number of reasons. But if your goal is losing weight or reversing diabetes or improving your cholesterol, eating cake conflicts with that goal. Those calories will produce the opposite outcome.

Can you imagine saying, "This is a special day! I'm going to go drop a brick on my foot"? No, of course not, that makes no sense at all.

But have you said, "This is a special day, let's get ice cream"? Or maybe you say, "This is a special day, let's treat ourselves." Yes, we make that kind of statement all the time.

You may be rolling your eyes and saying, "Oh, you're no fun, lighten up. I only do that once in a while."

I'm not encouraging you to stop eating indulgent food on occasion. I'm encouraging you to consider whether food needs to be part of your celebration and whether including it enhances your life or makes you feel frustrated and discouraged. Even though something wonderful happened, you don't need to eat food.

You don't need a special occasion to eat cake. Go ahead and eat whatever you want regardless of whether it is a special day. And celebrate life's events with cheers and high fives and hugs and jokes and smiles. You may find that by the time the cake comes around, you're already feeling full.

While We're on the Subject . . .

You may have heard the adage "The best way to predict the future is to create it."[5] We don't choose every circumstance of our lives, but we have more control over circumstances than we may think. So today, I ask you, "How do you know if you're having a happy holiday?"

This exercise has a few rules. First, you must be specific about what brings you joy during the holidays. The more detail you put into imagining the scents, flavors, and images of the season, the easier it'll be to find them.

Second, be realistic. You can't bring people back from the dead, and you have to exist in this dimension. But other than the laws of physics and the constraints of your resources, have at it.

Third, your happy holiday criteria must be self-generated. That is, nothing in your perfect scene can depend on someone else doing something. Waiting for other people to generate your happiness is a recipe for heartache and resentment.

OK, are you ready? Here we go.

Let's flip the calendar a couple of pages to January 1. Imagine sitting in your favorite place with a wonderful feeling of contentment wrapped around you like a blanket. Life is peachy. Gosh, that was a wonderful holiday. Now imagine someone sits next to you and asks, "How was your holiday?"

You say, "Wonderful," and then begin to paint the scene. What, specifically, made the day or the season so wonderful?

My mind calls up images of jingle bells on doorknobs, making treasured family recipes to share with others, decorating my home like we live in the Biltmore, and smelling cinnamon, orange, and clove simmering on the stove. I clink glasses with friends and family, witness the magic of the season through children's eyes, and indulge enough to feel fancy while still fitting into my jeans in January. If those things have happened by December 31, I feel good.

Other things make the holidays memorable too. Children being polite and gracious to their elders, no one getting sick, family members not discussing politics, no car trouble on the way to Grandma's, good weather, my husband buying the correct gift for me, my kids eating the fancy food I've made, my favorite music at church, short checkout lines at the stores, and delighted reactions to all the gifts I purchased for others, to name a few. But we've already discussed that.

Now let's zoom back in the calendar to the present day. You've painted that picture of the events that made you feel content, so make it happen! What will ensure that the elements which made you feel so happy take place? You've identified your priorities; now schedule them.

Make Your Own Rules

Start respecting the boundaries you set for yourself by being N.I.C.E.

N = Notice. Notice when you're approaching an internal boundary that needs to be respected. You wouldn't tell someone else that what they need is selfish and unimportant, so why is it OK to tell yourself that? Hearing negative self-talk signals that a boundary is in jeopardy. Feeling anxious, guilty, or otherwise overwhelmed are other signs that you aren't respecting one of your personal boundaries.

I = Identify. Verbalizing what you've noticed helps clear the mental clutter. Say something like, "I accepted a piece of cake I don't want to eat because someone offered it to me. I'm pushing my boundary of eating within my calorie needs because I feel obligated to eat food given to me." In doing so, you've noticed how you feel and why you feel that way, without judgment or evaluation. Wow! You're so evolved. Go you!

C = Commit. Once you notice how you feel and identify why, commit to respecting that boundary. "I'm committed to making choices that will support my health and vitality." That may mean saying no to people who made cake or saying no to another part of yourself, like the part that wants to stay up late watching TV instead of getting enough sleep to be energized for a morning workout. The commitment to respect your own boundaries doesn't mean putting yourself first at the expense of others; it means taking care of yourself so you can take care of others.

E = Engage. Act! Put your metaphorical foot down, steel your resolve, take a deep breath, and say, "Thanks, but I'm good." Turn off the TV and get in bed so you can wake up energized for exercise. Get off the couch and prepare a healthy lunch and snacks for the next day so you don't end up in the drive-thru lane at a fast-food restaurant. Do it. Nothing changes if you don't engage with your own commitment.

Reflect

1. What makes you feel content and happy?
2. How much of that is within your control to create?
3. What can you do this week to set yourself up for success?

WEEK 43

The Happy Grown-Up's Guide to Healthy Living

To be healthy these days, we're asked to follow so many rules: eat the right food, do the right workout, and wear the proper shoes. Have the right clothes, use the most current technology, write everything down, and log it in your activity tracker. And if you don't post your progress on social media, does it even count?

I'm going to tell you a secret. Are you ready? You don't have to do any of that to live a healthy, fulfilling life. You can break most of the rules and still come out ahead.

Rule #1 to Break: Wait Until You Know What You're Doing

A client recently expressed surprise when I revealed that she didn't have to run to participate in a 5K race. "I can walk?" she exclaimed. "I didn't know I could do it if I wasn't a runner!" Of course you can! You can walk, roller-skate, walk on your hands, and stop halfway to make a peanut butter sandwich if you want to. Just get out there and start moving. We can be self-conscious about whether we're making a fool of ourselves by doing things differently. But most people are so preoccupied with their own self-consciousness that if they notice what you're doing, they'll assume you're doing it correctly and they're the weird ones. Embrace the weird. You're allowed to be weird.

Rule #2 to Break: Assume One-Size Nutrition Advice Fits All

Nutrition advice changes as quickly as Tallahassee's weather, and while some fundamentals stand the test of time, not every new piece of research necessarily applies to everyone. Humans come in different shapes and sizes; we have different needs, preferences, and settings for our bodies. We can honor our personal truths without approval or permission from anyone else.

For example, in the span of one week, I read that Greek yogurt is one of the healthiest foods you can eat and that eliminating dairy is the solution to our obesity epidemic. Some of my friends have benefited from eliminating dairy from their diet, but I consider yogurt an excellent source of protein that makes me feel great. Remember: health and fitness articles are written for the average reader. You aren't average. You're awesome. Take the advice that makes sense to you and leave the rest for someone else.

Rule #3 to Break: Pretend You're as Stressed Out as Everyone Else

Have you been in a conversation where everyone is venting about how tired and busy they are, and you feel like you should commiserate and agree that everything's terrible even when you don't think it is? Stop! Just because everyone else runs themselves into the ground, chasing fads, and trying to be cool, doesn't mean you have to do that too. You can opt out of the crazy and choose to travel slower, more simply, and a lot happier and healthier as a result. Let everyone run circles around you trying to impress everyone else. The only person who needs to be impressed by what you're doing to manage your health is you.

If trying to keep up with the right way to be healthy is taking all the fun out of life, then throw out the rulebook, wish everyone good luck, and forge ahead on your own. Someone else may consider you weird, you may feel silly at first, and you may get a few questions or curious looks. Smile, wave, and enjoy the progress that comes from living healthy by your own rules. Give 'em something to talk about.

While We're on the Subject . . .

Not many people know this, but I can predict the future. I can state what will happen and, most of the time, be accurate. I can't predict lottery winners or the weather—nothing like that. My gift has been honed over years of listening, watching, and learning from people and how they live. I normally keep this skill a secret from others and use it only for my own purposes. But today I'll share some predictions with you. Specifically, I'll reveal which decisions you make will have the most staying power and the biggest impact on your life.

Are you ready?

Prediction: They will be challenging but rewarding. When you make a choice that sticks, it will be because you feel great about it. Habits and goals with the most longevity challenge you enough so you're looking forward to the end and then feel proud when you get there. I predict that your favorite decision this year will be one that pushes you just enough to be fun.

Prediction: It will include friends. Even the toughest battles are easier with a sense of community and teamwork. I don't need my crystal ball to know you'll love a life where you're part of a community that cares about you and cheers when you succeed. You'll keep going back.

Prediction: It will be worth it. You already know that establishing new routines takes discipline, time management, and an internal desire for the benefits. Even your favorite activity will feel like a chore sometimes. But it will feel worth it.

Make Your Own Rules

Write a list of what scares or intimidates you. Read the list aloud and notice where you feel tension in your body. Are you holding your breath? Does your stomach lurch? Do your shoulders rise toward your ears? Intentionally release your shoulders, let your jaw fall slack, and exhale. You have the skills to do more than you think. Choose the least intimidating item on your list and take action on making it less scary today.

Reflect

1. Think about a time a unique or brave decision worked out well. How did you feel when you made that decision?
2. Where in your body do you feel a reaction to making a brave choice?
3. What will be your next brave choice?

WEEK 44

Blast from the Future

Have you ever written a letter to yourself? One semester during my high school years, an English teacher told us to write a letter to our future selves giving advice or maybe a warning. Later in life, we were supposed to read the letter and draw some kind of conclusion. It's fun to read what a younger, more naïve version of yourself may have considered profound, sage advice and then compare how your life turned out to what your younger self predicted.

Maybe the reverse could also be meaningful. What would our future selves say if they could reach back to where we are now and give us advice? As a wellness coach, I often encourage clients to look around and see what's written on their walls. Hindsight is 20/20, and when we realize after a catastrophe that the signs were obvious, we could have saved ourselves a lot of time and headache if we had read what was written there.

Of course, we can't always predict the future, but we can draw a reasonable conclusion based on logic and common sense to determine whether our current situation will likely end well or otherwise. The signs are there: a growing list of medications, a doctor advising a lifestyle change, chronic fatigue, increasing forgetfulness, or feeling overwhelmed all indicate that our train is running off the rails. How many of these signs do we pass each day, planning to do something about them when life calms down, but ultimately ignoring them?

Countless books have been written on the lessons we learn over a lifetime: Don't sweat the small stuff. Forgive early and often. Buy the accident policy!

And, of course, we listen and nod and reflect on this wisdom, and then go on with our lives. The luxury of spending more time with family is easy for someone at the end of their life to suggest, when the practical application of that good advice is harder to achieve. Many things are easier said than done. Many of the smartest, wisest choices seem possible—if only. If only things were a little different, less hectic, less expensive, less inconvenient.

Reflect on your life up to this point. What advice would you give a younger version of yourself, knowing what you know now?

While We're on the Subject . . .

Have you ever noticed that, after time has passed, you're able to think about previous events objectively, without emotion? That means we have gained wisdom. When we recall past experiences and relive how we felt, we might as well be experiencing those events all over again. I'm grateful when I can look back on a painful time and not feel the same emotions again. That means that I've healed, moved on, and can see the situation more clearly. Learn from the past. Gain and use the wisdom.

Make Your Own Rules

Try some of these techniques for hearing the wisdom of your future self.

Ask for It. Close your eyes, connect with yourself, and listen. Listen for what your heart and soul are saying. In *Dead Poets Society*, Robin Williams's character tells the boys to lean toward the trophy case to hear the wisdom of the students who had come before them. Do that. Be still, close your eyes, ask yourself for advice, and listen. Then believe it.

Pretend You're Not Yourself. If listening to yourself seems weird, then pretend you're giving advice to someone. If a friend was headed on the path you're now walking, what would you say? And what would you not say for fear of hurting that person's feelings? Tell that to yourself in a kind way. Then believe it.

Write Your Own Ending. I was amazed by a story of a man who wrote his obituary in advance of his death and didn't like what it said. So, he tore it up and wrote a better one. Then he lived that life. A slight shift in habits can change the course of an entire life cycle; write a few drafts of your obituary and pick your favorite version. Then believe it.

Reflect

1. What does the writing on the wall of your life say?
2. What lesson could your younger self remind you of today?
3. Do you believe you can write a different ending to your life? Why?

WEEK 45

Balance Health Goals with Art and Science

The pharmacy where I worked as a teenager had a sign in the back displaying the store's hours of operation. You may have seen it in other businesses:

> We're open most days around 9:00 or 10:00. Occasionally as early as 7:00, but sometimes as late as 11:00 or 12:00. We're closed around 5:30 or 6:00. Occasionally as early as 4:00, but sometimes as late as 11:00 or 12:00.

The sign gives more exceptions to the rules and always makes me chuckle. The rambling list of possibilities sounds a lot like me when people ask whether their weight loss plans will work. Reducing calories and increasing exercise should work, but sometimes they don't. You may lose weight at first, then stop losing weight. You may do everything right, but some medical condition is causing a plateau. You and your friend may follow the same plan, and one experiences results but the other doesn't. Why? Losing weight is more of an art than a science.

Science is quantifiable. It's either right or wrong and can almost always be explained with facts, data, and reason. Science is using a food scale to measure your portions so you know exactly how many calories you eat each day. Science helps us manage our health, especially when we monitor our cholesterol, blood pressure, or blood sugar. Science gives us helpful statistics, such as how losing 10 percent of our body weight can reduce risk factors for heart disease. Science tells us how much insulin we need. Science plays a role.

Art, on the other hand, is open to interpretation. The same piece of art can be viewed differently by various people, just as a size 1 on one person feels as comfortable and manageable as a size 4 on someone else. Art is connected to our personal values, and when health is art, we can create a picture of what balance means for us. Health as art is about quality rather than quantity, about knowing that maintaining healthy habits will result in healthy returns, even if the numbers don't always add up. Art makes us whole.

Science plays a role and art makes us whole. We need both to make magic happen in the world of weight loss. Consider these balance points as you work on your goals of achieving a healthy weight.

Balance Calories with Consistency. I've maintained my current weight for about five years, but I still weigh my portions most of the time. Calorie management is a big part of weight loss, and attention to detail can be the difference between losing weight and maintaining it. But what's more important than the everyday ratio of calories in versus calories out is the consistent pattern of a deficit over time. Like watching the stock market or investing for retirement, performance over the long haul matters most.

Balance Your Weight with Your Waist. The science of weight loss tells us that 3,500 calories equals one pound of fat. So, using 3,500 calories through exercise and reduced calories should equal a pound of fat lost, right? Yes, it should. Except when it doesn't, which is usually about a week before you need to fit into a bridesmaid dress or rented tuxedo. Relax. So much of what happens inside your body can make those numbers on the scale go haywire. Medications, not drinking enough water, your current hormonal state, the workout you just finished, and what you ate for dinner last night all factor into the number on that scale. Your body is a living organism that fluctuates all day long. Put the scale away and focus on the waistband of your jeans instead. If it's changing, so are you, regardless of what that hunk of metal and plastic tells you.

Balance Perfection with Progress. I enjoy reading stories of people who faced immense odds or setbacks, figured out a way to overcome them, and later achieved epic levels of triumph. I often refer to these stories when clients are stuck in the muck of imperfection, thinking they'll never progress because every day something happens to push them back. That, my friends, is called life. Success is not found in everything going according to plan, but in finding a way to move forward despite setbacks. You don't have to get it right; you just have to get it going.

While We're on the Subject . . .

Weight loss isn't only a numbers game. Neither is it as simple as making better choices. Progress toward our health goals requires a combination of science and art, especially when the canvas is an ever-changing living organism that often plays by its own rules.

So relax. You've got this. Enjoy those days when all the elements of your healthy lifestyle come together and you knock the ball out of the park. Balance them with the days when you have to focus to make any ground. If you're consistent, your success story will become a work of art.

Make Your Own Rules

The next time you feel like you're hitting a brick wall, consider these signs of progress and healthy change:

1. You're consistently in a better mood.
2. Everyday tasks are easier.
3. You have more energy and yawn less.
4. You're more optimistic.
5. You feel stronger (and maybe even see muscle definition).
6. Someone else notices that you seem happy.
7. You're craving less sugar.
8. Your digestion is better.
9. You have an enhanced sense of well-being.
10. You can't explain why but you feel great.

Reflect

1. What is one of your favorite pieces of clothing or jewelry to wear?
2. How do you feel when you wear it?
3. What about that piece is representative of you?

WEEK 46

Curiosity Can Lead to Healthier Living

Ever since I was captivated by a painting in a fourth-grade school textbook, I've been fascinated by the domestic lives of colonial Americans. My mind often drifts to what life may have been like for the Pilgrims who arrived on the cold, stormy shores of New England in 1620. I love to read the diaries of colonial women and learn the mundane minutiae of their lives: the contents of their kitchens, the neighborhood drama, and the work involved in maintaining a homestead in the middle of the wilderness. I wonder how they felt when they stepped onto the shore of an unknown land with no concrete knowledge of what lay ahead. The beginnings of the United States may not have happened in the idyllic fashion we envisioned as children, but the stories arouse my curiosity and admiration because venturing into the unknown is courageous.

In a somewhat related note (trust me, this all comes together), I once heard a radio interview with Walter Isaacson, author of *Leonardo da Vinci*, a biography of the man esteemed as one of the most prolific creative geniuses of all time. While I listened and drove through the rural highways of south Georgia on my way back to Florida, I thought about the intelligence of a mind like da Vinci's and wondered if I'd ever experience thinking as nimble and creative as his. Then Isaacson made a point that gave me hope: da Vinci wasn't only brilliant, he was also curious. Yes, he crafted ideas from observations, but without the intense curiosity that made him constantly peel back layer after layer of everyday situations, his true brilliance might have remained just an admirable level of intelligence. I'm not brilliant, but I am curious. And while I admire intelligence, the courage to be curious is a trait I admire more.

Courage and curiosity come in handy as we pursue healthy living, especially during the holidays. We may not experience a breakthrough in our thinking about ourselves until we're willing to challenge the status quo or what we think are circumstances out of our control. During the holidays, more than any other time, people talk about traditions that must be followed, meals that have to be eaten, cookies that have to be baked. And I wonder . . . what if? What would happen if this was the year when the holidays were different?

I'm not saying change is essential. I'm asking whether we're curious enough to explore what would happen if the holiday season was different this year, even on paper. And maybe I'm asking if we have the courage to poke at our traditions and try something different, like da Vinci would.

Let's start with the first part: what would happen if your holiday habits were different this year? On a piece of paper, brainstorm what would happen if you didn't make as much food or didn't eat so-and-so's cheese dip or didn't open the next bottle of wine. What would happen if you didn't let the morning workouts go on hiatus until January? What could be good about that change? What could be annoying? You could even sort your brainstorming into a list of the pros and cons of a holiday season that was a little different. Allow yourself to be curious. You don't have to take action on anything; sometimes just knowing the possibilities is interesting.

Then, maybe something you wrote down seems significant. Something you might be curious enough about to try. Something you might have the courage to try. Something you might have the courage to try and be bad at. At least you tried. Leonardo da Vinci would have tried. Now you have something in common with Leonardo da Vinci. Not everyone can say that.

While We're on the Subject . . .

The courage to be bad at something new embodies the spirit of what made da Vinci a creative genius and what made it possible for the Pilgrims to step onto new ground. The courage to be curious enough to try something different is arguably the trait that leads to breakthroughs.

The holidays lie ahead of us, and we know what that means: many opportunities to maintain the status quo, to copy and paste the way things always are, or to challenge them through curiosity and courage. This week, slow down, examine your holiday surroundings, and ask, "What if?"

Make Your Own Rules

If curiosity isn't a natural inclination, try some of these exercises.

> **Snap a Pic.** Take a picture of something that captures your attention every day for seven days. At the end of the week, examine the photos. What do you notice?
> **Ask Questions.** Reach out to an elder and ask them to tell you stories from their childhood. What was school like? What was their first job? What is their most memorable, funny family story?
> **Schedule Unscheduled Time.** Set aside thirty minutes one day this week to wander outside. Take in your environment with an open mind and heart. Follow a bug. Study a leaf. Listen to the sounds . . . and wonder.

Reflect

1. What problem or opportunity are you facing right now?
2. What possible solutions have you come up with?
3. What would happen if one of those solutions worked?

WEEK 47

Let It Go for Thanksgiving

One of my favorite Thanksgiving traditions is having no Thanksgiving traditions. My family has some established must-do items for other holidays, but Thanksgiving is a wild card. We may be at the beach on Turkey Day. We've taken the Staten Island Ferry to see the Statue of Liberty on Thanksgiving, and for the past couple of years, we've gone camping.

It's liberating to not be tied down to certain things needing to happen for the day to feel right. A Thanksgiving dinner of cheeseburgers and a pint of beer at a diner or a pot of gumbo over a campfire? All good for my family.

Are you feeling stifled by your holiday food traditions? Challenging convention and rebelling against the expected can be a breath of fresh air.

Plenty of us feel obligated to eat everything presented to us on Thanksgiving. Some folks tuck their napkin into their collar, open their arms, and say, "Bring it on!" Others wring their hands because they don't want that I-can't-believe-I-ate-the-whole-thing feeling, but they also don't want to hurt someone's feelings or miss out on the tasty food they love.

Either way, let that guilt go. Thanksgiving is one day. Everyone says healthy living is a lifestyle, but not really. It's a series of small decisions over a long time. You don't have to commit to a healthy lifestyle to reap the rewards of good health.

That may sound like the opposite of what everyone has told you. Weight loss success stories are full of testimonials about how you toss the quick fix to the curb and adopt a healthy approach for your whole life. But that's not true.

You don't need to commit to being healthy for the rest of your life. You only have to commit to doing that today. Or at this meal. Right now. You deserve to feel great all the time, but if that's more than you want to think about, just feel great now.

Then, if you liked the feeling, make the commitment again. You can make healthy choices—the ones that keep your body feeling light, energetic, and mentally clear—all day long if you want to. Or you could stop and go back to the old way. You choose!

In a perfect world, you'd make one healthy choice, then another, and another until you look back and realize you're smack dab in the middle of a healthy lifestyle.

But let's not think about that right now.

When the holidays arrive, you've got old family recipes to make, relatives coming into town, suitcases to pack, and who knows what else. Adding exercising and watching what you eat on top of all those responsibilities may seem overwhelming. So don't. Just make the healthy choice today.

You don't have to stay tied to holiday traditions of eating too much and regretting it later. You can go to the beach or get on the ferry to see the Statue of Liberty. You can go camping. You can book a hotel room and watch TV all day. Whatever. You do you.

Thanksgiving is about reflecting on what we're thankful for. It's also about rebellion. After all, if the Pilgrims hadn't envisioned a better future, they wouldn't have sailed across the ocean. This year, rebel against convention. Throw that all-or-nothing approach out the window. Toss your holiday traditions to the side. Live healthy one moment at a time and be thankful for the right to do it.

While We're on the Subject . . .

This year don't worry about what you eat. Instead, focus on why, when, and where. By taking cues from our surroundings and environment, we can create healthier holidays that focus on family and friends, not food.

Why Am I Eating? It's no secret that we eat for reasons other than hunger. Celebrations, tragedies, anxiety, and boredom all send us to the pantry looking for something to distract us. On holidays, however, these triggers become amplified and seem more urgent than they would on any other Thursday. To make your holiday healthier, note why you're eating before you take a bite. Is your stomach growling, or did your house turn into Grand Central Station with the arrival of family? If you're not hungry, reconsider that nibble and instead focus your energy on taking deep breaths and drinking some water.

When Am I Eating? Eating every three to four hours keeps our metabolism humming and prevents a drop in blood sugar. However, hosting family gatherings often leaves little time for well-balanced meals and snacks. If you find yourself devouring a slice of pumpkin pie as soon as Aunt Betty begins critiquing your homemade stuffing or surviving on cheese and crackers laid out for holiday guests, call a time-out. Prepackage some sliced fruit or chopped vegetables with a healthy fat, such as whole, natural almonds, and stash them away. When you're hungry, that healthy snack will provide the energy and satiation you need to withstand the most jovial of holiday guests.

Where Am I Eating? Eating on the couch while watching football, eating while standing and socializing at a party, and eating in the car headed for Black Friday shopping will likely lead to consuming many more calories than you realize or need. Limit meals to the table. When you have to eat on the go, measure your portion and pack it ahead to ensure portion control. Staying fueled for holiday shopping is easy and guilt-free when you know your snacks are helping your body stay healthy, not adding unwanted pounds.

The holidays are full of delicious aromas, flavors, and time-honored recipes, all of which can be enjoyed with a focus on the psychology of food. By noting why, when, and where you eat, you can stay healthy through the holidays and enter the New Year minus one resolution.

Make Your Own Rules

Get Real about Special Food. We're lucky enough to live in a country where food is bountiful. We have 24/7 access to Walmart, which carries every vice you can eat. Sure, your mom only makes her special stuffing once a year, but what's to stop you from making it in the middle of July?

Instead of placing so much emphasis on the food traditions surrounding the holidays, create memories by interacting with your family in a new way that isn't food related. Institute an annual Christmas Day walk. Break out the puzzles and board games. Stage a family talent show. Focus on the people.

Profile the Threats. Speaking of people, know whom to look out for. Your mother-in-law, your coworker, or your neighbor—you know who it is. That person who corners you and insists you try the recipe made especially for you. I call these people "the feeders," and you can categorize them this way:

- The Nurturing Feeder needs connection and affection, which you can provide without eating pie.
- The People Pleaser wants to feel needed and appreciated, which you can provide by praising their thoughtfulness (but not eating the fruits of their labor).
- The Controlling Feeder wants to take you down. They may be angry that you aren't underwriting their bad habits, or they may be jealous of your discipline and subsequent success. Regardless, your best line of defense is to change the subject.

Learn to Say No Creatively. When you're confronted with something that's not on your plan, use positive language to redirect the attention away from your refusal to indulge. Be sure to respond with one or all of the following sentiments.

- Express gratitude: "Thanks for offering!"
- Acknowledge the effort: "So thoughtful of you to make these for me."
- Suggest an alternative: "I'm not hungry now, but I'll look for it later."

Reflect

1. What do you need right now?
2. What could be possible if you felt completely supported?
3. What would you do first in pursuit of a personal goal today?

WEEK 48

Embrace the Weirdness of Change

"I'll do better next time." "No one's perfect." "Well, at least it wasn't as bad as it could've been!" Is this you?

I love hearing people making these statements because they give me an opportunity to flip what sounds like a negative experience into a positive one. Hidden in each comment is positive energy and confidence in the possibility of a better future, even though the speaker probably feels like a failure. A positive attitude is essential in achieving our health goals and demonstrates the kind of resilience that characterizes successful people.

Resilience can be a crutch, though. These hopeful, optimistic statements may be the reason we don't ever make progress in our health because they strengthen our resistance to change. If you wonder why you keep deciding to do something unproductive to your health goals, while the healthier alternative is equally convenient, you aren't alone.

Change is hard, but most of us are up to the challenge. We encounter minor changes almost every day and navigate them with relative ease. Change usually stops us in our tracks, not when it's difficult but when it's uncomfortable.

Discomfort is painful. We want it to end. We want to return to that comfortable place where we knew the answers.

That's normal, and for some people, discomfort is a temporary condition, which ends when life calms down. For others, it's a pattern that becomes an obstacle to needed change. When you notice resistance to change as a pattern, one of these reasons may be the trigger.

- **You may not believe a better life is possible.** When all we know is failure and all we hear is criticism, imagining success is difficult, even when we crave something different. Being confident with change requires a certain level of expectation about what lies ahead, but often the only guarantee is that the outcome will be interesting. And that's not always comforting.
- **The pain of staying the same is more bearable than the pain of change.** We've all watched someone sink to the bottom of the pit of despair before he or she will accept help, and perhaps we've been that person. Even our most self-destructive habits can be a source of comfort. Sometimes we must admit that we don't want an outcome badly enough, and that might be OK for now.
- **The logistics of change may be overwhelming or guilt-ridden.** Wanting something to happen doesn't make it easy to achieve. Necessary commitments may be inconvenient at first or require a financial investment. We may have to set boundaries, which may involve other family members' cooperation. Sorting out these details takes work, but the effort pays off.

That uncomfortable time of committing ourselves to the new choice, even though we're unsure what's on the other side, is where we make the leap from "I'll do better next time" to "Wow, I did it!" Leaping into change may be the last thing you want to do. So, maybe you shuffle over to it or sit with it. If you want life to be different, you can start now.

While We're on the Subject . . .

Imagine two neighbors decide they want to build identical houses. They call a contractor to come and advise them, and as the contractor explains the construction process, one neighbor interrupts.

"Oh no, I don't want you to use nails on my house," he says.

The contractor is confused. "You don't want any nails?"

"No," the man answers. "Nails are a pain. I don't like them. I know other people who've built houses without nails, so I'm going to skip that part."

"Are you sure?" the contractor asks. "Nails are one of my most valuable tools. Every house I've built that satisfied a customer has included nails. Without them, you may not be happy with your house."

"I'm sure," says the man. "I don't want to deal with nails."

The contractor starts to construct the houses, and soon the man who wanted his house built without nails notices that his neighbor is moving in.

"Hey," he says to his neighbor, "why isn't my house done yet? The contractor started building them on the same day. We have the same kind of house. But you're moving in, and I'm still waiting. What gives?"

The neighbor pauses. "Yes, construction began on the same day, but you didn't want to use nails. That's your choice, but no nails means it'll take a lot longer to finish your house. I used all the available tools, so my house is done." And he went inside, sat in his favorite chair, and enjoyed his new house.

In my work as a health coach, I often hear another version of this story. Many people have a weight loss goal, but as we discuss the various tools and processes involved, some of them stop me and say, "No, I don't want to do that part."

They may not want to omit empty calories from alcohol or soda, log foods in a journal, or eat smaller portions. Those choices are hard, and they've heard about other people who lost weight without making those changes, so they want to skip them.

And that's fine. You can certainly achieve a weight-loss goal without doing what other people rely on for success. But frustration sets in when your progress is slower than expected. Friends who decided to use all the available tools may reach their weight-loss goals faster and maintain them longer, like the neighbor who moved into his house first.

We have all the tools sitting around us, waiting to be used in pursuit of our goals. The tools exist because others have discovered they work well. If you're struggling to make progress while others sail past you, they may be using tools you've ignored.

That's OK. The tools are always there, and you can reach into the toolbox anytime and pick up a nail.

Make Your Own Rules

Does picking up a new tool feel weird? Are you resistant to considering new outcomes? Try this exercise for flowing with fear.

Ask yourself, "What about this makes me afraid?" Listen to your answer, and gently notice what happens with your body. Ask yourself, "And then what?" Continue this process with awareness and compassion until you reach the answer that speaks to you. Fear is only a feeling, and it's trying to tell you something. Listen.

Reflect

1. If you were your own best friend, what advice would you give yourself today?
2. What three words describe your life right now?
3. What three words do you want to describe your life right now?

WEEK 49

Aim to Stay the Same During Times of Stress

As a health and wellness coach, I come across two general categories of folks: those who strive to maintain self-care and healthy habits through stressful phases and those who don't.

If you've been working to make changes in your health, I raise my coffee mug to you and make eye contact in a significant way, because a healthy lifestyle is hard work. Congratulations! As a reward for your perseverance and commitment, you now advance to the next level of changing your life: staying the same.

Yes, you read that correctly. In the previous chapters, I've talked about how to create positive, healthy change. Now I'm shifting course and encouraging you to stay the same. But this is advanced-level work because there are times of the year when just maintaining the status quo is going to be a significant accomplishment!

Achieving a goal of staying the same starts with identifying what that means. What do you want to maintain? For some, that means staying in the same clothing size; for others that means sticking to an exercise program, no matter what. When life gets wonky, going for a run is a priority because I can tell the difference all day long in my stress levels. What do you want to maintain?

After you decide, ask yourself why. Why is that goal important? Why bother? Can you think of a time when you regretted not doing it? When have you met the goal and said, "That was worth the effort"? Connect with why this is important because that knowledge will be helpful in the next step.

Now, look at the calendar to identify times when this goal is vulnerable. My work schedule often involves travel, and while running is a portable activity, my commitment seems to wane when I'm not at my house in my own routine. I'm committed to the benefits of running, so when I've let the habit lapse, I regretted it. I know what I'm missing if I let that happen again. I need to decide what's necessary to maintain the habit despite travel and whether I'm willing to do that.

The good news is that you know how to do this. Your calendar may be different, and your schedule may be busier, but you're the same person, and you're in charge. You'll need an increased level of commitment, and you'll have additional opportunities to slip, but you know how to stick to your plan.

While We're on the Subject . . .

I'm repeating this phrase because it's important: *whether I'm willing to do that.* Remember what I said about being able, willing, and ready in Week 37?

Sometimes what looks good on paper and seems like a worthy accomplishment is a goal we know we don't care enough about to work for. That's OK. This is optional. But if you want to survive a stressful time and feel glad that you maintained your healthy habits, have a head-to-heart conversation about what you're willing to do to make that happen.

Make Your Own Rules

Celebrate your hard work with these (mostly) calorie-free treats under $15:

- Download a new song for your workout playlist or book for your e-reader.
- Reserve quiet time for yourself to do something you don't usually get to do.
- Take a nap.
- Put a dollar amount for each benchmark reached into a vacation account.
- Find a beautiful coffee mug or teacup so you can start each day with a piece of art.
- Buy fresh flowers for your kitchen as a reminder that it's a place where beautiful habits can bloom.
- Buy a frivolous magazine and read it (not while standing in the grocery store checkout lane).
- Have your clothes professionally altered to fit your more svelte self.
- Purchase a new kitchen tool to enhance your healthy cooking.
- If you choose to reward yourself with food, splurge on the gourmet version of something you already buy regularly, such as your favorite brand of coffee or a bottle of wine.

Reflect

1. What have you overcome during the last few months that makes you feel proud?
2. What's going well in your life right now?
3. What are you most excited about trying next?

WEEK 50

Choose New Year's Goals Wisely

Do you typically make resolutions or goals at the beginning of the year? If so, they probably fall into two categories of excitement. Some goals and plans you're ready to tackle, excited to pursue, and feel prepared for. Your confidence is high that you'll accomplish them, and you're eager to start.

Other goals you're not quite as enthusiastic about. They might be carried over from year to year, like a knickknack you received as a gift and think you should display even though you don't care for it. These goals might begin with the words "I should" or "Hopefully, I will." You can see the value of the outcome, but you're not that into it. Your confidence is low that this will happen, but you'd be happy if it did.

Does that sound like you? If so, come with me. We'll examine these two goals more closely and, ultimately, I'll encourage you to consider abandoning one. Let's start with the first one.

The goal you're excited about is the one you're certain you'll achieve. Why are you so confident? What assures you that this'll be a slam dunk? Don't skip this part with a wimpy answer like "I just know." Think deeply about why this year is the time to take action, what experiences have brought you to a place of readiness, and why you're the person to take this on. Write your answer down and read it. This is a powerful affirmation about where you'll focus your energy in the coming year. Exciting!

Now, put that goal down and pick up the second one, the one you feel like you should do or hope will happen. This one is also important and valuable, but you aren't as confident that you'll pull it off. Why? What experiences make you feel doubtful or ambivalent? Are you missing a skill or strength that prevents you from feeling more ready to tackle it? What would need to happen for this goal to feel more like the first one? Write all of that down too.

Then, take the second list and poke at the questions a little more. Can you acquire that skill or strength? Are you willing to make the necessary changes so the path to success is straighter? Is there anything about working on this goal that excites you a little bit?

If your answers are no or even if they're ambivalent, I challenge you to put down that goal and turn your attention to where you're saying yes. As our lives become busier, louder, faster, and more stressful, the health implications of living in the fast lane mount. Stress leads to more cardiovascular disease, sleep disorders, and higher anxiety, all of which are like poison. One step we can take in a different direction is to simplify our lives, connect with what brings us joy, and focus energy on something that can go well.

Earlier I said that I would challenge you to abandon one of your goals, but I was only saying that to be dramatic. I don't want you to abandon it, but I encourage you to choose wisely where to invest your energy. Go where you can win. Start there and give yourself time and space to evolve into the person who's prepared and excited to take on the other goal, which will wait patiently for you.

While We're on the Subject . . .

But what if that second goal is something you need to do? Am I saying you're off the hook because working on it doesn't bring you joy? No. I'm saying that the energy you put into it at a low level of confidence will be wasted if you could be putting energy into something that will be successful. Here's why: as you succeed in the tasks where you have the most confidence, those secondary goals may become more appealing. Success breeds success. Start where you can succeed, and what you can succeed at will expand.

Make Your Own Rules

Starting where we can succeed can seem daunting. If you're not sure what that goal is, discover it by keeping an energy journal.

- At the end of each day, make a list of the tasks that consumed your time—everything from work to play to family stuff to errands. Write it all down.
- Look at the list and sort the items by whether they drained your energy or boosted your energy.
- Review the list again and rank them according to how much they drained or boosted your energy.
- Finally, look at the outcome of each activity. What was the best use of your time? We can't always spend our time on the activities that boost energy, but if we start there, we have more enthusiasm for the tasks that don't.

Reflect

1. If you could be anyone else for a day, who would you be?
2. What is it about that person's life that is appealing?
3. If you were your own loving parent, what would you do for yourself today?

WEEK 51

Bend in the Winds of Change

I watched a good portion of Hurricane Michael blow through Florida's Panhandle from my front porch. As a lifelong southerner, I've seen a few tropical storms and hurricanes, and I'm stuck between standing in awe of nature's power and wanting to give it a wide berth to show my respect. This storm was no different, and as I sipped my coffee and wondered when we'd lose electricity, I sat under the cover of my porch and watched the trees.

A lot of pine trees surround my house—some big fat ones and some little spindly ones. I placed my bets on which would survive and which wouldn't. As the bands of wind and rain came through, the trees swayed. And when they began to bend, I went inside and moved to the window.

As I watched the trees bend, I thought about their root system. I wondered how far the roots went down and how far a pine tree could bend. Was it better to be a big fat tree or a little skinny tree? And I noticed some admirable tree traits.

A while ago, I saw a quote by Jim Rohn with a picture of a tree that said, "If you do not like life's circumstances, move. You are not a tree."[6] The words made me feel kind of bad for trees because they can't move away from their circumstances. They have to stand there and take it, whether the adversity is a drought or a Category 4 hurricane.

We're like that sometimes too. If circumstances are bad, someone may say, "Well, if you don't like it, then leave." Other times, we're rooted where we are, either by family or obligations or other life situations. Picking up and leaving isn't a viable option. Like a tree, we have to stand there and take it.

A lot of people feel that way about their health. They need to make changes, and sure, someone can say, "Well, just eat better. Just get up earlier and exercise. Just quit buying cigarettes. Just do it." But some people are rooted in lives that can't be undone that easily, and they feel like they have to stand there and take it.

But as I watched the trees in the storm, I realized they were doing more than standing there. They were swaying, bending, and releasing. Even when we're rooted where we are, we can do that too.

Sway When You Can. The storms of life push us around, but we don't have to just stand there. Like a tree, we sway throughout our lives to allow for this event or that unexpected change of plans. These times can make us stronger, more cognitively nimble, and more creative. Sway when you can so your self-care habits continue, even in a storm. Swaying might mean compromising on when you exercise rather than stopping altogether.

Bend When You Need To. As I watched the trees bend, I thought about how stubborn and committed they were to withstand so much pressure and not fall over. Their resilience reminded me of when life gets so hectic that if we want to stay healthy despite the chaos, we need to make even bigger compromises. We may let exercise go and focus on eating healthy. If food choices are out of our control, we can counteract the extra calories by staying active. Bending in this way means we might not be getting everything we need, but at least we're getting some of it. And sometimes that's enough.

Let Some Branches Fall. Those trees swayed and bent, but they also released some branches to stay upright. This is a loss, for sure, but one that's regained over time. Don't be afraid to let some branches fall off your tree if it means you stay rooted in what supports your physical and emotional health. New branches will grow; the loss is temporary.

After the storm, we clean up. And as we reach out to help our neighbors recover, our roots will go deeper, and we will be stronger. If another of life's storms is headed your way, be like a tree. Sway, bend, release, and hang on to your roots.

While We're on the Subject . . .

Sometimes we may need to stop, look around, and take a few steps back to see the mess we've made before we can start cleaning it up. If food feels like a mess these days, simplify by prioritizing, organizing, and compromising.

Grumbling about not getting everything you want is OK, but that doesn't change anything. Know what you're willing and not willing to let go of to feel your best.

Make Your Own Rules

Prioritize What You Want. You've likely heard the phrase "begin with the end in mind," right?[7] That's good advice because it demands purpose for your actions. The first step to figuring out how to eat healthy is to decide what eating healthy means to you. Do you want to eat more vegetables? Drink less soda? Eat fewer meals in restaurants and more at home? Lose weight? Knowing this helps simplify your process because you can focus on meeting a specific goal and choose actions that support it.

Next, think through the to-do list of what it will take to achieve the goal. Let's say your goal is to eat more vegetables. That seems like a simple objective, but you may need to write out the steps to make that happen:

- I want to have more vegetables in my diet, so . . .
- I need to decide what meals and snacks I can incorporate vegetables into, so . . .
- I need to buy the groceries. That means . . .
- I need to go to the store or order the food to be delivered. Then . . .
- I need to make time to do any necessary preparation to follow through.

Going through this process helps you notice the next step: being honest about the obstacles to your goal. Maybe you look at that list and think, yeah right, I don't have time for that. Maybe you have a friend who often invites you to your favorite burger place for lunch. Maybe eating vegetables is something you feel like you should do but don't want to. You owe it to your future self to be honest about what you want and what's standing in your way so that later on you'll have a good answer when your future self asks why you didn't do something sooner.

Once you've come to terms with all of that, decide what you're willing to do (or not do) to achieve the outcome you want. This could mean adding vegetables to meals three days a week rather than every day. Maybe you're so motivated that you're ready to try a meatless day once a week. This is where the rubber meets the road. You've identified what you want, so how much hassle are you willing to put up with to get it?

Get Organized. All right, you just did a lot of work, and I told you this would be simple. The rest is easier, I promise.

Being organized about your food means taking the necessary steps to make healthy food as convenient as junk food. You're more likely to eat fruits and vegetables if they're the first item you see in your refrigerator. Get them out of the crisper drawers and into a bin—front and center. Take the extra step to chop and package snacks to go, or spend a little more for the precut veggies and remove that time barrier. Learn from the days you don't reach your goal and ask, "How can I win next time?" Then, do it!

Be Ready to Compromise. Food can be healthy or cheap or tasty. You can choose two. You have to compromise! Eating healthier may mean scrimping on other things so you can spend more on quality food. The healthiest meal for you may not taste like Grandma's macaroni and cheese with two sticks of butter and the crackers crumbled on top. Choose your two priorities and remember that future self.

Reflect

1. If my body could talk, it would say . . .
2. I feel most energized when . . .
3. Today I will . . .

WEEK 52

Make Time for Dreaming

In a 1961 episode of *The Twilight Zone* titled "A Penny for Your Thoughts," a man is given the gift of mind reading after a penny lands on its edge. He's astounded by what goes on inside people's minds, especially when he overhears his coworker conjuring up nefarious plans of how to rob their employer and retire on the riches. But as the episode progresses, the mind reader learns that the coworker's thoughts are innocent, indulgent daydreams—not plans for a robbery.

That story came to mind recently when I mentally wandered to a scenario I felt was a waste to think about because it could never happen. But as I snapped back to reality, I remembered that some of the most fantastical daydreams can become the inspiration for a daydream's more mature and sophisticated older sister: vision.

When we make goals for improving or changing any area of our life, it's important to know the difference between dreaming about change and planning for it. Those who create sustainable, satisfying change move beyond the daydream and create a vision supported by progressive goals and action steps. That doesn't mean daydreaming is a waste of time. Both visions and daydreams are important exercises for balanced health. Today, I challenge you to explore your daydreams and determine whether anything in them is calling out to become part of your reality.

Fantastical daydreams are fun to indulge in. Imagining an experience that you never intend to fulfill gives your brain a break. I consider these daydreams the equivalent of splurging on a dessert after a long period of disciplined nutrition choices. They let our brains get their wiggles out, play a little, and recharge without disrupting our lives.

Sometimes, though, elements of these mind escapes have a little more pull to them. Just as every joke contains an element of truth, some daydreams hold an element of yearning. If we pay attention to the underlying themes of daydreams, we can uncover opportunities to set goals to bring desired elements into our day-to-day life. For example, the man who daydreamed of robbing his employer and retiring on a cash windfall may have no intention of breaking the law, but he does yearn for a comfortable retirement. Can you see how that daydream might turn into a life goal?

When you notice that your daydreams have elements of true desire, take those parts down from your mental cloud and put them on paper in a structured wellness vision. A vision is the big picture of what we want to achieve down the road. Whether that's a few months, a year, or longer, you should aim for a time frame that you can easily reach but is more challenging than you can achieve in a few weeks. A wellness vision keeps us grounded and focused, and it serves as that happy place to go to in our daydreams when the work of achieving it becomes tiresome.

A vision has elements that distinguish it from a simple goal or a daydream. Put your dreams to the test and see if they're ready to be part of your real life.

A Vision Is Based in Reality. The first criterion for a vision is you must be able to make it happen. Stealing money without consequence and retiring comfortably is an unlikely outcome in real life, but planning for a comfortable retirement is within reach. Your vision should be something that can happen independently of anyone else's choices or actions. Thinking "if only so-and-so would . . . then I could . . ." is a sign that your vision is unrealistic. Enjoy the daydream of so-and-so doing what you wish they would and move on.

A Vision Is Exciting and Bold. Even though your vision needs to be grounded in reality, challenge yourself and think big. Your vision should make you wonder about whether you can achieve it. It should give you goosebumps. Go ahead and admit what you want. Wanting something isn't necessarily selfish or wrong. If you had no obstacles and were guilt free, what would you do with your life?

A Vision Requires Work You're Willing to Do. Once you admit what you want and put it through the "could this happen" reality check, decide what you're willing to do to achieve it. And it's OK to acknowledge that you value and appreciate something but have other higher priorities to work toward right now. Yes, you can want something, know it's possible, feel it's important, and know you'll be glad you achieved it, but still not act on it. That unwillingness may indicate the desire rightfully belongs in the category of daydream for now. When you want it bad enough to take action, it belongs in your vision.

Have you ever planned a beach vacation in midwinter and felt like you could smell the sunscreen and hear the seagulls? That's a palpable vision. Think about what an ideal day would be like. When you close your eyes and imagine yourself living that way, you should be a little surprised when you open them and you're not there. You should also feel more excited to work on it because it's so possible to you.

A Vision Doesn't Have to Wait. A vision becomes real to us when we live in it. I encourage my clients to create a vision they can participate in immediately. If you envision living an active life where you participate in community races and have eliminated the need for medication, start attending weekend events and participate at the level you're ready for. You can be in your vision now by achieving mini goals that move you toward the vision you've created.

Pay attention to your daydreams. Some are whimsical flings of the mind, but others are calling to you. Listen. Pull them down from your mind cloud and see if they're ready to be part of your real life.

While We're on the Subject . . .

I wrote this book because I care about you, and I want to be part of the positive life you create. You've made it this far. You've done the work and allowed yourself to dream about what could be, and I'm proud of you. Congratulations! Now go and get it.

Make Your Own Rules

Are you ready to write a vision statement?

Your vision statement is what you imagine your life can and will be. Creating and, most importantly, using a vision statement keeps you focused on your goals and helps you avoid distractions.

Step 1: Look at the big picture of what you want to create for your life.

- Your vision statement is the starting place for your goals.
- It helps you take a daydream and make it reality.
- It reflects what your life and career is about.
- It is your happy place.
- It is layered with behaviors, actions, strengths, feelings, values, and relationships.
- It should give you confidence, energy, and a feeling of authenticity.

Step 2: Get specific about what outcomes you want to enjoy.

- What kind of person do you want to be?
- What specifically do you want to accomplish?
- What types of habits do you want to have?
- Why is this worth the work you will put in?
- What character traits do you have that will give you an edge?
- What kind of challenges should you prepare for?
- Where can you turn for help when you need it?

Step 3: Use the template below to get started.

In my wellness vision, I am _____, _____, and _____.

I _____ daily to _____ because _____.

I enjoy _____, which is a benefit of my commitment to _____.

As a result, I am now _____.

When things get tough, I know I can _____ and _____.

Values, Strengths, and Supports

Every day is not easy, but I know I have the tools I need to be successful.

Reflect

Try one of these visioning exercises:

- **Postcards from the Future.** Write a letter to yourself from your vision. What's it like there? What does "a day in the life of you" look like? What happened to get you there?
- **The Movie Set.** Imagine I've sent a camera crew to do a documentary on you. But I can't be there, so you need to describe yourself so they can find you. Where will you be? What will you be doing? How will they know it's you?
- **The Rocking Chair.** Fast-forward to when you're ninety years old, sitting in a rocking chair on the front porch, and telling the stories of your life. What was your proudest moment? What was worth working hard for? How did people describe you? What were you glad you did?

Notes

1 "What Oprah Knows for Sure about Finding the Courage to Follow Your Dreams," Oprah.com, accessed August 31, 2021, https://www.oprah.com/spirit/what-oprah-knows-for-sure-about-finding-your-dreams#:~:text=The%20whole%20point%20of%20being,if%20you%20weren't%20paid.

2 Mao, Jun J, Qing S Li, Irene Soeller, Kenneth Rockwell, Sharon X Xie, and Jay D Amsterdam. "Long-Term Chamomile Therapy of Generalized Anxiety Disorder: A Study Protocol for a Randomized, Double-Blind, Placebo- Controlled Trial." Journal of clinical trials. U.S. National Library of Medicine, November 2014. https://www.ncbi.nlm.nih.gov/pmc/articles/PMC5650245/.

3 Mary Beth Faller, "Bob Bowman Uses Michael Phelps to Explain How to Achieve Excellence," ASU News, January 30, 2017, https://news.asu.edu/20170130-sun-devil-life-bob-bowman-uses-michael-phelps-explain-how-achieve-excellence.

4 Qtd. in Conor Heffernan, "Changing Household Cooking: Jack LaLanne and the 1950s," Physical Culture Study, September 4, 2017. https://physicalculturestudy.com/2017/09/04/changing-household-cooking-jack-lalanne-and-the-1950s/.

5 This adage is often attributed to Abraham Lincoln, but variations of this adage are attributed to several other people, including Alan Kay. David Sivak, "Fact Check: Did Abraham Lincoln Say, 'The Best Way to Predict the Future Is to Create It'?," Check Your Fact. checkyourfact.com, July 24, 2019, https://

checkyourfact.com/2019/07/24/fact-check-abraham-lincoln
-best-way-predict-future-create/.

6 "You Can Change, You're Not a Tree," YouTube, accessed
September 28, 2021, https://www.youtube.com/watch?v=tQBcc
OpnM6M.

7 "The 7 Habits of Highly Effective People," Franklin Covey,
accessed September 3, 2021, https://www.franklincovey.com
/the-7-habits/.

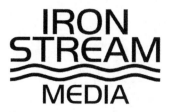

IRON STREAM MEDIA

If you enjoyed this book, will you consider sharing the message with others?

Let us know your thoughts. You can let the author know by visiting or sharing a photo of the cover on our social media pages or leaving a review at a retailer's site. All of it helps us get the message out!

Email: info@ironstreammedia.com

 @ironstreammedia

Brookstone Publishing Group, Iron Stream, Iron Stream Harambee, Iron Stream Fiction, Iron Stream Kids, and Life Bible Study are imprints of Iron Stream Media, which derives its name from Proverbs 27:17, "As iron sharpens iron, so one person sharpens another." This sharpening describes the process of discipleship, one to another. With this in mind, Iron Stream Media provides a variety of solutions for churches, ministry leaders, and nonprofits ranging from in-depth Bible study curriculum and Christian book publishing to custom publishing and consultative services.

For more information on ISM and its imprints, please visit IronStreamMedia.com

 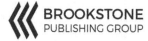